Inside...

The Quick-to-Read Tips
That Can Give You Big Results!

LOSE THE **BUTT,**
LOSE THE **GUT**
AND GET OUT OF
THE RUT!™

"Almost" Effortless Ways to Get You
Looking and Feeling Better Again

Robert Wolff

Published by The Creative Syndicate

LOSE THE **BUTT**, LOSE THE **GUT** AND GET OUT OF **THE RUT!**™

"Almost" Effortless Ways to Get You
Looking and Feeling Better Again

Robert Wolff

Published by The Creative Syndicate

10400 Overland Road, Suite 143
Boise, Idaho, USA 83709

Copyediting by Lynette Smith
Book Interior Design by Betty Abrantes

Book Information: www.RobertWolff.com

Print edition ISBN: 978-1-937939-06-9
Electronic edition ISBN: 978-1-937939-07-6
First printing 2002, Second Printing 2012
Library of Congress Control Number 2011961675

Note: Inspirational quotations not otherwise attributed were written by
Robert Wolff.

INTRODUCTION

Lose the Butt, Lose the Gut and Get Out of the Rut!

A name you'll remember with tips you won't soon forget.

In this crazy non-stop, on-the-go world, it's little wonder so many of us have so little time to take better care of ourselves.

Then when we do, we overdo it. And if we don't, we end up feeling guilty about not doing enough of the things we keep telling ourselves we should.

Enough already!

It's time for something different, something fresh and something so simple to add to your life, that it's going to feel *almost* effortless.

What you're about to discover are the weekly tips—those small little things that can only take seconds—that have the power to make profound changes in how you look and feel.

Now imagine a full year—yes, *52 weeks*—of brand new weekly motivational, exercise and nutrition tips, just waiting for you to use.

Lose the Butt, Lose the Gut and Get Out of the Rut! takes the guesswork out of how you can look and feel better, by giving you the tips that work.

This book gives you what you need to change your body and motivate and inspire you at the same time.

You're going to find its Weekly Quick Tips for motivation, exercise and nutrition will give you a complete year's guide for simple, easy changes you'll see and feel beginning the first week.

One of the biggest reasons people hold back from changing how they look and feel—and maybe you've been one of those people—is the belief that exercise, eating right and staying motivated takes too long or is too difficult and demanding.

Not true.

Lose the Butt, Lose the Gut and Get Out of the Rut! gives you tips that are brief, powerful and positive.

Each of these 156 tips has been carefully selected to fit easily in your lifestyle, regardless of your available time or experience level.

In addition to the book's Weekly Quick Tips, you'll also find a Weekly Guide that allows you to chart your progress regarding the changes you'll see and feel—from the physical to the emotional.

You'll find the power of such reinforcement—every week seeing and feeling, firsthand, how your life and body are changing—to be highly motivating.

You'll experience this power anytime you want to turn the pages back to the previous weeks and read the notes you made about the changes you saw and felt taking place in your body and life.

You'll smile when you see just how quickly and how far you've come.

Lose the Butt, Lose the Gut and Get Out of the Rut! is the Daily and Weekly Guide that will give you what you desire: a fast, simple way to change how you look and feel in only minutes each week.

Robert

CONTENTS

ROBERT WOLFF

1
WEEK

Quote of the Week

Where the mind goes, the body follows.

THIS WEEK'S MENTAL TIP

One disciplined action will bring you many rewards. To prove this, let's say you've taken the action to eat healthier foods. Just by that one action...

1. Your body now has more energy because of the healthy foods you are eating.

2. You feel better and not so sluggish.

3. Your digestion has improved.

4. You sleep better.

5. Your skin complexion has improved.

6. You're saving money because, on average, it costs you less to eat healthy foods than processed and junk foods.

7. You're getting leaner each week—losing the fat and keeping your lean muscle tissue—because you're now eating foods containing the proper ratio of protein, carbohydrates and fat.

8. And because you're feeling and looking better, your appearance is improving, thereby raising your self-confidence, self-image and self-esteem.

9. All of this helps improve your relationships with others, as well as your job performance, and it raises your belief in yourself that you can set goals and achieve them.

10. And because you see and feel the results from doing just *one* disciplined action of eating more nutritiously, you now have a strong desire to begin an exercise program, which will change your body and the way you feel, even quicker. And this will give you even more rewards.

THIS WEEK'S EXERCISE TIP

To tighten glutes and legs while walking and without exercise equipment, try lengthening the stride of your walk and to make it more aerobic, really swinging those arms up and down, forward and backward. By taking longer steps, you activate more glute, quad and hamstring (back leg) muscle; and as you know, a well-worked muscle quickly becomes a well-toned and attractive-looking muscle.

THIS WEEK'S NUTRITION TIP

When buying tuna in spring water, always check the label. Fat content—even from the same company and the same brand—can vary substantially. The reason? Tuna caught closer to the shore are leaner (less fattier foods in their diets) than tuna caught farther out to sea (more abundant sea life and higher fat diets). Don't believe me? Just go to the store and *sea* for yourself.

1

The Little Things I Did This Week
To Help Me Reach My Goal and
Change My Body and Life

For Nutrition: _____

_____

_____

_____

_____

_____

_____

_____

_____

For Exercise: _____

_____

_____

_____

_____

_____

_____

_____

_____

The Little Things I Did This Week
To Help Me Reach My Goal and
Change My Body and Life

1

For Thinking Differently: _____

_____

_____

_____

_____

_____

_____

_____

_____

To Help Inspire Myself: _____

_____

_____

_____

_____

_____

_____

_____

_____

1

The Little Things I Did This Week To Help Me Reach My Goal and Change My Body and Life

The Changes I Can See: _____

_____

_____

_____

_____

_____

_____

_____

_____

The Changes I Can Feel: _____

_____

_____

_____

_____

_____

_____

_____

_____

2

WEEK

Quote of the Week

Every year I live I am more convinced that the waste of life lies in the love we have not given, the powers we have not used, the selfish prudence that will risk nothing, and which, shirking pain, misses happiness as well. No one ever yet was the poorer in the long run for having once in a lifetime 'let out all the length of the reins.'

—Mary Cholmondeley

THIS WEEK'S MENTAL TIP

One of the easiest ways to change how you feel is through the power of affirmations. Simply tell yourself what you want to experience—for example, in weight loss, you'd say something like "I look and feel great at ____ pounds"—and keep repeating it at various times throughout the day; early morning and late evening are best. Affirmations activate the unconscious section of the mind—the real powerhouse that changes your life—by giving it new commands upon which to act. The key to making affirmations work is that they must be positive and always stated in the present tense; as if you've already achieved that change in your life right now.

THIS WEEK'S EXERCISE TIP

Drink plenty of water before doing any exercise. Research has shown that for every 1% of weight your body loses from dehydration (i.e., loss of water), your peak performance can drop by 10%.

THIS WEEK'S NUTRITION TIP

For a more restful sleep, try eating some carbohydrates about 90 minutes before bedtime. The reason? Carbs help boost *serotonin* levels in the body; *serotonin* helps the body relax and is one of the three neurotransmitters commonly known as "the feel good hormones." Just don't eat too many. Like any nutrient, too many carbs, especially before bedtime, can make you fat.

2

The Little Things I Did This Week To Help Me Reach My Goal and Change My Body and Life

For Nutrition: _____

_____

_____

_____

_____

_____

_____

_____

_____

For Exercise: _____

_____

_____

_____

_____

_____

_____

_____

_____

The Little Things I Did This Week
To Help Me Reach My Goal and
Change My Body and Life

2

For Thinking Differently:
_____
_____
_____
_____
_____
_____
_____
_____

To Help Inspire Myself:
_____
_____
_____
_____
_____
_____
_____
_____

2

The Little Things I Did This Week To Help Me Reach My Goal and Change My Body and Life

The Changes I Can See:

_____

_____

_____

_____

_____

_____

_____

_____

The Changes I Can Feel:

_____

_____

_____

_____

_____

_____

_____

_____

3

WEEK

Quote of the Week

There is only one thing that will really train the human mind and that is the voluntary use of the mind by the man himself. You may aid him, you may guide him, you may suggest to him, and, above all else, you may inspire him. But the only thing worth having is that which he gets by his own exertions, and what he gets is in direct proportion to what he puts into it.

—Albert L. Lowell

THIS WEEK'S MENTAL TIP

To keep progressing when others have stopped, always change your program. Never do the same thing twice. This will help spike your metabolism and helps keep your body off-guard so it never quite gets the chance to habituate and become stale. Not only that, but it keeps you motivated and looking forward to your next workout because you're always doing something new and different.

THIS WEEK'S EXERCISE TIP

For incredible looking calves, one of the best exercises you can do is without weights, equipment or in a gym. It's your stairs. Without shoes on, simply place the balls of your feet (the top 1/3 of your foot) on the edge of the stairs. Keeping your knees locked, allow your heels to lower below the stair, then, raise your heels up above the stairs as high as you can. Do this movement non-stop until you begin feeling a burning sensation in your calves. Stop for 15-25 seconds, then do it again two more times. After you've finished all three sets, lower your heels all the way down and stretch your calves by staying in this position for 30-50 seconds. Expect to be sore the next day or so. Repeat the exercise only when you can no longer feel any soreness. In 30 days you'll be happy at the changes.

THIS WEEK'S NUTRITION TIP

To lose weight, try this simple, but very effective European secret that spas and retreats have used for years. Chew your food *20* times before swallowing. Twenty times, that's all, and you'll be amazed at how something so simple could be so effective. Not only will your food take longer to eat—which will give your brain a more accurate and quicker message from the stomach that you're getting full—but properly chewed food is actually digested easier and its nutrients are used more effectively by the body.

3

The Little Things I Did This Week To Help Me Reach My Goal and Change My Body and Life

For Nutrition: _____

_____

_____

_____

_____

_____

_____

_____

For Exercise: _____

_____

_____

_____

_____

_____

_____

_____

The Little Things I Did This Week
To Help Me Reach My Goal and
Change My Body and Life

3

For Thinking Differently: _____

_____

_____

_____

_____

_____

_____

_____

_____

To Help Inspire Myself: _____

_____

_____

_____

_____

_____

_____

_____

_____

3

The Little Things I Did This Week
To Help Me Reach My Goal and
Change My Body and Life

The Changes I Can See:

_____

_____

_____

_____

_____

_____

_____

_____

The Changes I Can Feel:

_____

_____

_____

_____

_____

_____

_____

_____

4
WEEK

Quote of the Week

Be content with what you have;
never with what you are.

—B.C. Forbes

THIS WEEK'S MENTAL TIP

Stay sensitive to feedback. While exercising, keep your mind focused on your body and listen to what it tells you during and after each exercise. Are your muscles in tune with and feeling the movement? Does it feel like you're in the groove and moving like a well-tuned machine? Or is your body telling you to change things because it's not feeling what you're doing? Even in the middle of a set or exercise, don't be afraid to stop and try something else. Find the thing that your body wants you to do for it that *day*, that *hour* and that *minute*. Your body is a living, dynamic organism that's *constantly* changing every day throughout the day, and it's always talking to you. Keep your mind focused on it and you'll hear it loud and clear.

THIS WEEK'S EXERCISE TIP

Looking for a great aerobic and anaerobic workout but short on time? Easy. Do more in less time; that's the secret for fitness success. During your workout, simply decrease your rest time between exercises and sets to no more than *35* seconds. The combination of exercise and less rest time increases heart rate, amps metabolism, gets blood pumping throughout your body and floods your body with those wonderful natural opiates (the "feel good hormones") called *endorphins*.

THIS WEEK'S NUTRITION TIP

To make skim milk taste more like regular milk, put it in the freezer 15 minutes before drinking. The colder the milk, the more rich it tastes. And speaking of skim milk, if you want to increase your daily protein intake—which helps firm muscle tone—try adding fortified skim milk powder to yogurt, cottage cheese, soups, and desserts. Not only is it a terrific nonfat protein source, but you'll get all the benefits of the extra power-packed protein your body needs, and you won't even taste the difference.

4

The Little Things I Did This Week To Help Me Reach My Goal and Change My Body and Life

For Nutrition: _____

_____

_____

_____

_____

_____

_____

_____

_____

_____

For Exercise: _____

_____

_____

_____

_____

_____

_____

_____

_____

_____

The Little Things I Did This Week
To Help Me Reach My Goal and
Change My Body and Life

4

For Thinking Differently: _____

_____

_____

_____

_____

_____

_____

_____

To Help Inspire Myself: _____

_____

_____

_____

_____

_____

_____

_____

4

The Little Things I Did This Week To Help Me Reach My Goal and Change My Body and Life

The Changes I Can See: _____

_____

_____

_____

_____

_____

_____

_____

The Changes I Can Feel: _____

_____

_____

_____

_____

_____

_____

_____

_____

5
WEEK

Quote of the Week

Did you ever hear of a man who had striven all his life faithfully and singly toward an object, and in no measure obtained it? If a man constantly aspires, is he not elevated?

—Henry David Thoreau

THIS WEEK'S MENTAL TIP

One of the most powerful techniques to change your body and your life is through visualization. But, if you really want fast results, add the power of *feelization*. Like the name implies, *feelization* is where you actually feel—*through your imagination*—what it would be like to actually be 10 pounds lighter or have flatter abs or tighter glutes and thighs. In essence, when you imagine how your body will feel—*a preview*—before you actually reach that goal, it helps propel your unconscious mind that much faster to the fulfillment of your desired result.

THIS WEEK'S EXERCISE TIP

To tone waist and side abdominal area, do trunk twists with a broom handle. Place and hold the wooden handle on your shoulders with it resting on the base of your neck; either seated or standing, twist from side to side, non-stop, for 2-5 minutes. To avoid a thick waistline, stay away from using weights. Many people who have used weights for side abdominal work report easy muscle gains that have thickened their waistline, but extreme difficulty in trying to lose the muscle while trying to get leaner. Unless you want a more-or-less permanent addition of muscle and a bigger waistline, stick with the broomstick.

THIS WEEK'S NUTRITION TIP

Looking for a simple trick to raise the good cholesterol (HDL) in your body? Simple. Do at least *10 minutes* of aerobic activity like walking, biking or any other exercise that gets your heart and lungs pumping.

5

The Little Things I Did This Week To Help Me Reach My Goal and Change My Body and Life

For Nutrition: _____

_____

_____

_____

_____

_____

_____

_____

For Exercise: _____

_____

_____

_____

_____

_____

_____

_____

_____

The Little Things I Did This Week
To Help Me Reach My Goal and
Change My Body and Life

5

For Thinking Differently: _____

_____

_____

_____

_____

_____

_____

_____

To Help Inspire Myself: _____

_____

_____

_____

_____

_____

_____

_____

_____

5

The Little Things I Did This Week To Help Me Reach My Goal and Change My Body and Life

The Changes I Can See:

_____

_____

_____

_____

_____

_____

_____

_____

The Changes I Can Feel:

_____

_____

_____

_____

_____

_____

_____

_____

_____

6
WEEK

Quote of the Week

We can accomplish anything we feel the urge to do. We all have within us the capacity to achieve what our souls desire. It all depends on the extent of our will power, and our ability to sacrifice unimportant things for the all-important goal. This alone is the measure of our achievement. No obstacles are too great. No matter what our past mistakes may have been, no matter how the false years may have misled and neglected us, it is never too late to start anew, never too late to attain to that complete expression of the self which alone makes for richly contented living.

—Stanwood Cobb

THIS WEEK'S MENTAL TIP

Always remember the mental principle of *The Last Deposit*. This principle states that your mind always remembers more strongly, the last experience of anything you do. That's why when it comes to your workouts or exercise, always make sure you end your training/exercise session by doing something positive like that extra rep, extra effort or anything else that leaves you feeling good about yourself. It'll be the first thing you remember when it comes time for your next exercise session.

THIS WEEK'S EXERCISE TIP

To elevate your metabolism and speed fat burning, try jumping rope. In fact, you don't even need a rope. Simply place your feet together, begin moving your arms like you are swinging a jump rope and start jumping up and down. And you don't need to jump high; an inch or so works great. Just keep the momentum going by jumping up and down and do this 20-30 times. Rest 20-35 seconds and do another 20-30. Rest 20-35 seconds and do one more set of 20-30 jumps. After your third set of 20-30, check your pulse rate and you'll feel it beating faster, you'll be sweating a little (maybe even a lot) and feeling great. For best fat burning results, do it at least 15 minutes *before* breakfast.

THIS WEEK'S NUTRITION TIP

After a workout, drink a can of diluted fruit juice. Try mixing ½ can of seltzer or carbonated water with ½ can of fruit juice. Not only will you reduce your calories by 50%, but it will help your body better absorb the carbohydrates in the fruit juice to replenish muscle fuel (glycogen) it used during your workout. And it tastes great!

6

The Little Things I Did This Week To Help Me Reach My Goal and Change My Body and Life

For Nutrition: _____

_____

_____

_____

_____

_____

_____

_____

For Exercise: _____

_____

_____

_____

_____

_____

_____

_____

_____

The Little Things I Did This Week
To Help Me Reach My Goal and
Change My Body and Life

6

For Thinking Differently: _____

_____

_____

_____

_____

_____

_____

_____

_____

To Help Inspire Myself: _____

_____

_____

_____

_____

_____

_____

_____

_____

6

The Little Things I Did This Week To Help Me Reach My Goal and Change My Body and Life

The Changes I Can See:

_____

_____

_____

_____

_____

_____

_____

_____

The Changes I Can Feel:

_____

_____

_____

_____

_____

_____

_____

_____

7

WEEK

Quote of the Week

As soon as you trust yourself,
you will know how to live

—Johann Wolfgang von Goethe

THIS WEEK'S MENTAL TIP

Use the power of momentum. The hardest thing for many people is just getting started, especially when it comes to exercise and eating better. One of the laws of physics states that an object will stay at rest until it's acted upon by an outside force. Let's change that to say *"A body will stay out of shape and lethargic until it's set into action by an inside force."* That means changing those self-limiting thoughts and beliefs and taking action. Just do a *little* something each day in the direction of making your body stronger and healthier. Just one little action, that's all. This sets in motion the power of momentum; and make no mistake, momentum is awesomely powerful. If you were to place a couple of 2 x 4s under the wheels of a 60-ton locomotive, you'd keep it from moving. But, once you remove those blocks and let the train start moving and gaining momentum, it will crash through a wall of concrete 10 feet thick! That's the power of momentum, and it's time you use that very same power to change your body and life.

THIS WEEK'S EXERCISE TIP

Looking for an easy way to work and change the appearance of those outer and inner legs? When doing that next set of leg exercises or any other leg exercise, simply change your foot position and feel the difference. To work more outer thigh, keep feet close together and pointing straight in front of you. For inner thigh, turn feet outward. For both foot positions, always be sure your knees travel in a straight line over your big toes.

THIS WEEK'S NUTRITION TIP

For better digestion, try having a piece of papaya before your meals. Papaya contains an enzyme called *papain* that helps break down the proteins in the foods you eat and helps your body better use the nutrients you give it. For many people, a slice of tomato or pineapple works well too.

7

The Little Things I Did This Week To Help Me Reach My Goal and Change My Body and Life

For Nutrition: _____

_____

_____

_____

_____

_____

_____

_____

_____

For Exercise: _____

_____

_____

_____

_____

_____

_____

_____

_____

The Little Things I Did This Week
To Help Me Reach My Goal and
Change My Body and Life

7

For Thinking Differently: _____

_____

_____

_____

_____

_____

_____

_____

_____

To Help Inspire Myself: _____

_____

_____

_____

_____

_____

_____

_____

_____

7

The Little Things I Did This Week To Help Me Reach My Goal and Change My Body and Life

The Changes I Can See: _____

_____

_____

_____

_____

_____

_____

_____

The Changes I Can Feel: _____

_____

_____

_____

_____

_____

_____

_____

8

WEEK

Quote of the Week

People who are unable to motivate themselves must be content with mediocrity, no matter how impressive their other talents.

—Andrew Carnegie

THIS WEEK'S MENTAL TIP

It's been said that with patience and persistence, one can achieve anything. But to be persistent, you've got to be motivated; and if you're like many people, that can be a tough thing to be. Here's a little trick that will help you stay motivated to change how you look and feel. Each day on a little Post-It note, write down one reason you want to look and feel different, and tape it to a sheet of paper. Do the same thing each day for 21 days. Look at yesterday's reasons and all the previous reasons first thing in the morning and last thing at night before bed. Thinking of new reasons will get easier with each day you do this. At the end of 21 days you will feel some huge changes inside—thinking, believing and acting differently—that will change your body and life. And whenever *you* feel a bit less motivated, simply look at all the reasons *you* wrote why *you* want this for *your* life, and that'll put you back on the right road again and keep you there.

THIS WEEK'S EXERCISE TIP

Looking for a great facelift you need only do once a week, one you can do anywhere in less than 60 seconds, and one that will keep your face and neck looking young and vibrant without surgery? You've found it, and it's called "the jaw extension." This great exercise works wonders for the neck and face, and it couldn't be easier to do. Simply keep your neck up and head erect. With the biggest smile you can make, tense your neck at the same time. Now, hold both in that position for 10 seconds then release for only 1-2 seconds and do it again for another 10 seconds. Repeat until you've done it six times. Do this only once per week and watch what happens.

THIS WEEK'S NUTRITION TIP

When it comes to nutrition, one size doesn't fit all, but here's a tip that seems to work very well for lots of people. Many have found that simply adjusting the time of day they eat carbohydrates greatly affects their body weight. The key, it seems, is to eat most of your high-carbohydrate foods early in the day (e.g., morning through 1-2 p.m.), then taper them down; and from early afternoon through the evening, do just the opposite you did in the morning and make most of the foods you eat protein. Many say their bodies more effectively use the carbs for energy early in the day as compared to eating them later in the day or at night. So remember this carbohydrate formula: *Most in the morning, less in the afternoon, least at night.* Do a bit of experimenting to see how it works for you.

8

The Little Things I Did This Week To Help Me Reach My Goal and Change My Body and Life

For Nutrition: _____

_____

_____

_____

_____

_____

_____

_____

For Exercise: _____

_____

_____

_____

_____

_____

_____

_____

The Little Things I Did This Week
To Help Me Reach My Goal and
Change My Body and Life

8

For Thinking Differently: _____

_____

_____

_____

_____

_____

_____

_____

To Help Inspire Myself: _____

_____

_____

_____

_____

_____

_____

_____

_____

8

The Little Things I Did This Week To Help Me Reach My Goal and Change My Body and Life

The Changes I Can See: _____

_____

_____

_____

_____

_____

_____

_____

_____

The Changes I Can Feel: _____

_____

_____

_____

_____

_____

_____

_____

_____

9
WEEK

Quote of the Week

*Nothing in life is to be feared; it is only
to be understood.*

—Marie Curie

THIS WEEK'S MENTAL TIP

So true. Fear is one the biggest reasons people don't achieve what they dream of or say they want. Yet fear is something that doesn't exist in the outer world; only in your mind. Has fear kept you from looking and feeling your best? When you were born, you came into this world with only two fears: the fear of falling and the fear of loud noises. Every other fear you have or have had has been learned. And if the fear of not knowing how you'd feel with a better looking body or the fear of not knowing what to do to get it or the fear of what if you aren't successful on "this diet" or "this workout" has kept you from taking any action, it's time to let go of those fears today. You'd be absolutely amazed at just how many people who look and feel great today had the same fears as you—and many, many times, worse fears than you. It's true. We all have had fears of one kind or another in our lives. And it's when you let go of them and let go of the way it's been, that you then begin, that moment, to experience the way it *can* be.

THIS WEEK'S EXERCISE TIP

Here's a great way to turn your driving time (for example, while sitting at a stop light) into a mini-workout; one that will do good things for your chest, shoulders and arms. You'll be using a principle called static contractions that has been shown to produce excellent results quickly. To work your chest, while keeping your arms straight out in front of you, place the *inside* of your wrists against the *outside* of the steering wheel in the 10 and 2 or 9 and 3 positions. Don't grip the wheel. Now try squeezing the steering wheel and hold that squeeze for 6-10 seconds. Release and repeat two more times. For shoulders, simply do the opposite; place the *outside* of the wrists on the *inside* of the steering wheel and push out (opposite of squeezing) and hold for 6-10 seconds. Release and repeat two more times. For arms, place both palms of your hands under the steering wheel and tense the biceps. Hold this position for 6-10 seconds. Release and repeat two more times.

THIS WEEK'S NUTRITION TIP

Many people—especially women—are deficient in iron. They feel tired and run down and wonder why. Lack of iron can be one of the biggest reasons. One of the best sources of iron, along with its other B vitamins, is molasses. Molasses is made from the residue left from making sugar out of sugar cane, and just a little of the stuff can do wonders for your energy and health. Try adding a little of it to muffins, waffles and whole grain breads. One tablespoon of molasses (depending on the kind) can provide up to 75% of your recommended daily iron allowance.

9

The Little Things I Did This Week To Help Me Reach My Goal and Change My Body and Life

For Nutrition: _____

_____

_____

_____

_____

_____

_____

_____

For Exercise: _____

_____

_____

_____

_____

_____

_____

_____

The Little Things I Did This Week To Help Me Reach My Goal and Change My Body and Life

9

For Thinking Differently: _____

_____

_____

_____

_____

_____

_____

_____

To Help Inspire Myself: _____

_____

_____

_____

_____

_____

_____

_____

9

The Little Things I Did This Week To Help Me Reach My Goal and Change My Body and Life

The Changes I Can See:

_____

_____

_____

_____

_____

_____

_____

_____

_____

The Changes I Can Feel:

_____

_____

_____

_____

_____

_____

_____

_____

_____

10
WEEK

Quote of the Week

Men are all alike in their promises. It is only in their deeds that they differ.

—Jean-Baptiste Moliere

THIS WEEK'S MENTAL TIP

Perhaps one of the biggest ways you lose power in achieving your dream—be it changing your body or anything else—is to tell others what you plan to do. Many years ago, I found that internal momentum creates external action, and the more momentum I created on the inside, the faster my plans on the outside would become reality. Then I discovered why that worked. Think of all the things you want to accomplish much like that of a big pressure cooker. For that cooker to work like it's designed, it must build up enough steam power. It's the same way for you. If you tell too many people too early what you're planning to do, your internal pressure cooker loses steam and it seems to take forever, if ever at all, to reach your dream. However, if you have enough steam, as in letting the excitement build inside you and keeping your secret silent, it fires your engine to want to achieve your goal quicker and quicker, with more focus and determination. Sure, you're so excited inside to tell everyone about it; yet, by keeping your dreams, goals and desires inside yourself until you've achieved your heart's desire, you keep the momentum fire burning hot and bright until you actually reach it. Try it, and you'll see exactly what I mean.

THIS WEEK'S EXERCISE TIP

Traveling and staying in a hotel no longer has to be bad for your body if you know some of the tricks to working it on the road. Here's a great one for legs, butt, calves and heart. Forget the elevator and find the stairs. Part one is the stride and works front and back legs and butt. Just like lunges or step aerobics, take one leg at a time and step up to next higher step. Then do the other leg up. Repeat non-stop for 15-20 times. If one step is easy, then go for two or three steps at a time. Now here's where things get good. Part two of the stair workout will work inner/outer thighs and butt. Instead of going up the stair(s) with front body facing forward like you did in part one, you'll be doing it sideways for the left and right sides. Go for only one step at a time since your lateral (sideways) motion ability will not be as flexible as your forward and backward movement. Be sure to work both legs equally for equal results.

THIS WEEK'S NUTRITION TIP

Here's a great all-natural stress and tension reliever that's ages old, yet very few know about. Mix one teaspoon of sage leaves (known as nature's sleep helper), one tablespoon of rosemary leaves (known as nature's tranquilizer), one ounce of dry peppermint leaves (known as nature's digestive). Mix everything and keep in an airtight container (like Tupperware). Boil water and use one heaping teaspoon of mixture to one cup of boiling water. Allow mixture to sit for about one minute in the cup of hot water and strain into fresh new cup. Add honey to sweeten and drink with small sips. Talk about relaxing mind and body *au naturale*.

10

The Little Things I Did This Week To Help Me Reach My Goal and Change My Body and Life

For Nutrition: _____

_____

_____

_____

_____

_____

_____

_____

_____

For Exercise: _____

_____

_____

_____

_____

_____

_____

_____

_____

The Little Things I Did This Week To Help Me Reach My Goal and Change My Body and Life

10

For Thinking Differently: _____

_____

_____

_____

_____

_____

_____

_____

To Help Inspire Myself: _____

_____

_____

_____

_____

_____

_____

_____

_____

10

The Little Things I Did This Week To Help Me Reach My Goal and Change My Body and Life

The Changes I Can See: _____

_____

_____

_____

_____

_____

_____

_____

The Changes I Can Feel: _____

_____

_____

_____

_____

_____

_____

_____

_____

11
WEEK

Quote of the Week

He who is silent is forgotten; he who abstains is taken at his word; he who does not advance falls back; he who stops is overwhelmed, distanced, crushed; he who ceases to grow greater becomes smaller; he who leaves off, gives up; the stationary condition is the beginning of the end.

—Henri-Frederic Amiel

THIS WEEK'S MENTAL TIP

There's a rather unspoken law of nature that says either you're growing or you're dying; there's no in-between. Look at the leaves on the trees. In the fall, the dead ones begin falling from the trees to make room for the new ones that will appear in the spring. Each year and every year this event happens with unfailing accuracy. Nature doesn't deviate her ways for anyone or anything, and it's the same for your body, mind and spirit. Inside you is a very powerful desire to learn and experience new things and grow in all areas of your life. Listen to your heart's desire for change and growth, and you find a sense of deep fulfillment and happiness. Refuse to hear and follow its call, and you feel unfulfilled. Each day, do just one little action to make your body look and feel better, and nature will reward you bountifully.

THIS WEEK'S EXERCISE TIP

Who said you can't have a great quick body tone-up at work or school? You sure didn't hear it here, because I'm about to give you a great one for your lower stomach. Simply sit on the edge of your chair or desk. Keep your upper body erect and knees close together. Lift the knees up just a few inches and really feel it work your lower stomach area. Only a few inches is all you need. Slowly lower the legs a few inches and repeat. Do this as many times as you can, then rest 20-35 seconds and repeat two more times. Now say "Bye-bye!" to that paunchy lower stomach.

THIS WEEK'S NUTRITION TIP

Looking for a great mid-morning/afternoon pick-me-up snack but don't want to spend a lot of money? Look no further than the bagel. In a study, the bagel was tested against many of those convenient but high-priced energy bars to see which one was better for athletes looking for energy. Guess which won? Did I hear someone say bagel? That's right, for much less than 50% the cost of that bar, you can have a nutritious bagel (pick your favorite kind) that many have found gives them more energy and lasts longer.

11

The Little Things I Did This Week To Help Me Reach My Goal and Change My Body and Life

For Nutrition: _____

_____

_____

_____

_____

_____

_____

_____

_____

For Exercise: _____

_____

_____

_____

_____

_____

_____

_____

_____

The Little Things I Did This Week To Help Me Reach My Goal and Change My Body and Life

11

For Thinking Differently: _____

_____

_____

_____

_____

_____

_____

_____

To Help Inspire Myself: _____

_____

_____

_____

_____

_____

_____

_____

11

The Little Things I Did This Week To Help Me Reach My Goal and Change My Body and Life

The Changes I Can See: _____

_____

_____

_____

_____

_____

_____

_____

_____

The Changes I Can Feel: _____

_____

_____

_____

_____

_____

_____

_____

_____

12
WEEK

Quote of the Week

We have more ability than will power, and it is often an excuse to ourselves that we imagine that things are impossible.

—Francois De La Rochefoucauld

THIS WEEK'S MENTAL TIP

How you look and feel has nothing to do with how you *can* look and feel. Did you get that? Your life and experiences thus far have nothing to do with all the possibilities that are available and waiting for you to experience. Today, I want you to do one little exercise or nutrition thing that you usually don't do. It could be something as quick and easy as drinking an extra glass of water or using fat-free salad dressing instead of your usual higher fat kind, or maybe it's trunk twisting 20 times from side to side or squatting up and down 10 times. Whatever it is, just do something different today and you will have broken through the familiar comfort zone (translation: *The Rut*) and will have caused a change inside you that will use more of your ability and release more of your willpower—power and ability you have yet to discover.

THIS WEEK'S EXERCISE TIP

Well, I never thought I'd be saying it to you, but it's time to throw in the towel. Uh, bath towel, that is. As in wrapping that bath towel around both door handles of any door in your home (or on the road) and doing a great exercise for your back. Place the door so that you're looking at the inside (thinnest part of the door (where the dead bolt sticks out) of it. Grab each end of the towel and wrap the middle of the towel around both of the handles. While holding both ends of the towel, step back until the towel is taut. With a slight bend to your legs and your body upright, lean back away from the door and with only your arms, pull your body close to the door then allow it to lean back again. Do this non-stop for 8-12 times, then rest for 20-35 seconds and repeat two more times. This is a great exercise that will tone both arms and back.

THIS WEEK'S NUTRITION TIP

How about some energy that will stay with you for hours and is actually good for you? Try adding beans, which are rich in complex carbohydrates and will also help reduce LDL (the bad cholesterol) in your body.

12

The Little Things I Did This Week
To Help Me Reach My Goal and
Change My Body and Life

For Nutrition: _____

_____

_____

_____

_____

_____

_____

_____

_____

For Exercise: _____

_____

_____

_____

_____

_____

_____

_____

_____

**The Little Things I Did This Week
To Help Me Reach My Goal and
Change My Body and Life**

12

For Thinking Differently: _____

_____

_____

_____

_____

_____

_____

_____

To Help Inspire Myself: _____

_____

_____

_____

_____

_____

_____

_____

12

The Little Things I Did This Week To Help Me Reach My Goal and Change My Body and Life

The Changes I Can See:

_____

_____

_____

_____

_____

_____

_____

_____

_____

The Changes I Can Feel:

_____

_____

_____

_____

_____

_____

_____

_____

13
WEEK

Quote of the Week

You've no idea what a poor opinion I have of myself—and how little I deserve it.

—W. S. Gilbert

THIS WEEK'S MENTAL TIP

What does your image project to yourself and the world? It's been said that what you are speaks so loudly to the world that they can't hear what you're saying. Meaning, how your body looks is like a giant billboard that flashes its neon sign brightly for all to see: "Look at me!" Your body and how you carry yourself tells the world, but most importantly it's a mirror to yourself, just how you feel about yourself on the inside. A fat, out of shape, lethargic body speaks the message loud and clear that you have a poor opinion about yourself and that eating right, exercising and taking care of your body and mind aren't important because you feel undeserving of such. But, change a few of those poor eating habits, start thinking *thin* thoughts, become more active and your body, your life and the new message it sends out for all to see will begin to change things in your life that will amaze you.

THIS WEEK'S EXERCISE TIP

Remember when you were in school and you saw the teacher writing on the blackboard and the underneath of his/her arm would jiggle? That was from flabby triceps, and it'll be something you'll never have to worry about once you do this exercise. It's called the dumbbell triceps kickback, and I'll take it a big step further by teaching you a trick that uses gravity. Take a light dumbbell in one hand. With a slight bend at the knees, bend your upper body forward until it's at about 90 degrees (i.e., bent over your legs). Place the upper arm holding the dumbbell against your side and bend your elbow so the dumbbell hangs down. Keeping your upper arm in the same position, bring your hand and dumbbell back behind you until your arm is fully locked out. Feel it in the triceps (back of the arm)? You bet, but just wait. Do the same thing again, only this time, raise your upper arm higher so that your elbow is above your back (compared to how you were doing it with it just resting against your side). Now kick (extend) the dumbbell back until the arm is straight. Wow! Yeah... what a difference a few inches against gravity makes. Do three sets of 10-15 reps for each arm.

THIS WEEK'S NUTRITION TIP

Want a couple of drinks that can help you live longer? Green tea and red wine may be your answer. Studies have shown that polyphenols—powerful antioxidants found in red wine and green tea—help fight cell damage from free radicals.

13

The Little Things I Did This Week
To Help Me Reach My Goal and
Change My Body and Life

For Nutrition: _____

_____

_____

_____

_____

_____

_____

_____

_____

For Exercise: _____

_____

_____

_____

_____

_____

_____

_____

_____

The Little Things I Did This Week To Help Me Reach My Goal and Change My Body and Life

13

For Thinking Differently:

_____

_____

_____

_____

_____

_____

_____

To Help Inspire Myself:

_____

_____

_____

_____

_____

_____

_____

13

The Little Things I Did This Week
To Help Me Reach My Goal and
Change My Body and Life

The Changes I Can See:

_____

_____

_____

_____

_____

_____

_____

The Changes I Can Feel:

_____

_____

_____

_____

_____

_____

_____

_____

14
WEEK

Quote of the Week

God will not look you over for medals, degrees or diplomas, but for scars.

—Elbert Hubbard

THIS WEEK'S MENTAL TIP

Some of the toughest battles you'll ever face in life are with yourself. The job you wanted that didn't come through and how you beat yourself up mentally about it. Or maybe it was all the pain and suffering you may have faced or are still facing by all the failed diets and workout plans gone wrong. Maybe it was the lack of motivation to "stay with the program" or how hard you pushed yourself to experience success this time and show all your family and friends that "this time" you were serious, only to have things go wrong—again. Yet life has a way of neutralizing and healing those pains, and it's called time and experience. All those experiences taught you some very valuable lessons that getting in shape is not about competition, comparison or proving anything to anyone else. It's about doing it because it makes *you* look and feel good. Because it's good for *you*, healthy for *you* and can help *you* live longer to experience and enjoy much more of the precious gift of life. It's about becoming the person *you*, and no one else, want *you* to become and doing things in your *own* way and in your *own* time, that feels best for *you*. Always remember that those in this world who achieve greatness in any calling are those with deep scars and even deeper happiness.

THIS WEEK'S EXERCISE TIP

Lots of people work in and visit the city. If you're one of them, you're about to learn how to get a fabulous little workout that will shape and tone your lower legs and thin that hard-to-work ankle area, simply by standing on the curb. While waiting for the light to cross the street, the trick is to place only your heels on the curb while allowing your toes to touch the street pavement, then raising the front of your shoes up above curb level (or as high as possible) and doing it for reps. These reverse-type toe raises are the secret to bringing out the best of your lower legs and will really help reduce ankle size at the same time, thereby giving your legs fantastic shape and appearance without even going to the gym. Do this each day and watch what happens in just 10 days.

THIS WEEK'S NUTRITION TIP

Looking for a bag full of memory boosting? Look no further than the produce section in the grocery store. Have a baked potato. It's loaded with memory-enhancing vitamin B6.

14

The Little Things I Did This Week
To Help Me Reach My Goal and
Change My Body and Life

For Nutrition: _____

_____

_____

_____

_____

_____

_____

_____

_____

For Exercise: _____

_____

_____

_____

_____

_____

_____

_____

_____

_____

The Little Things I Did This Week To Help Me Reach My Goal and Change My Body and Life

14

For Thinking Differently:

_____

_____

_____

_____

_____

_____

_____

To Help Inspire Myself:

_____

_____

_____

_____

_____

_____

_____

14

The Little Things I Did This Week To Help Me Reach My Goal and Change My Body and Life

The Changes I Can See: _____

_____

_____

_____

_____

_____

_____

_____

_____

The Changes I Can Feel: _____

_____

_____

_____

_____

_____

_____

_____

_____

_____

15
WEEK

Quote of the Week

*It is by attempting to reach the top in a single leap
that so much misery is caused in the world.*

—William Corbett

THIS WEEK'S MENTAL TIP

Perhaps one of the toughest things about life is how hard we are on ourselves to make it easier. Not content to take small baby steps towards our goals and dreams, we jump headfirst into things with everything we've got, hoping to skip many steps that are needed not only for our growth, but for the goals' completion. You've no doubt heard about or maybe even experienced this when people start exercising again. Instead of starting off slow, finding your groove and allowing your body to adjust, how many times have you done too much, over-exercised, gotten too tired or too sore and quickly become unmotivated to go through that again? Made you miserable, didn't it? We've all done it, so at least we're in good company. Next time, try this: Do only enough exercise that feels good to your body, but no more. Simply stop, even if you know you can do more. Next time, do a little bit more and stop again. Keep doing this until you've reached just the right amount of exercise for the right amount of time for your body and goals. You've got the rest of your life to enjoy looking and feeling great. No need to do it all in one day.

THIS WEEK'S EXERCISE TIP

Ever wanted to move more gracefully and quickly, with more speed and power? A fun way to start is by doing the fencing shuffle. And no, you won't need special clothes or sword. The fencing shuffle mimics the moves of what you'd see fencers doing as they move back and forth and side to side. This is also a great way to help strengthen leg muscles and connective tissue, and it will help increase agility and lateral stability. Begin by standing straight up with a slight bend to the knees. Place your right or left foot forward (whichever feels more natural). Raise your heels to put more of your bodyweight on the balls of your feet (the front of the feet

86

just before your toes). Move your body forward by using only the momentum of your body's leaning forward and springing off your toes. Your feet should come off the ground only a few inches as you move forward. Try going forward 6-12 inches and then springing back. Do the same thing to your left and right side and then come back. Begin by going only a few inches, and then increase the distance you move forward or backward and side to side as you get used to the movement.

THIS WEEK'S NUTRITION TIP

Are you a beef lover looking for the leanest cuts you can buy? Go for the round cuts such as round tip, top round, bottom round, eye of round, top loin, sirloin and lean ground beef. And when it comes to ground beef, buy the darkest color the store, has since the darker the red color, the leaner the beef will be.

15

The Little Things I Did This Week To Help Me Reach My Goal and Change My Body and Life

For Nutrition: _____

_____

_____

_____

_____

_____

_____

_____

For Exercise: _____

_____

_____

_____

_____

_____

_____

_____

The Little Things I Did This Week
To Help Me Reach My Goal and
Change My Body and Life

15

For Thinking Differently: _____

_____

_____

_____

_____

_____

_____

_____

To Help Inspire Myself: _____

_____

_____

_____

_____

_____

_____

_____

15

The Little Things I Did This Week
To Help Me Reach My Goal and
Change My Body and Life

The Changes I Can See: _____

_____

_____

_____

_____

_____

_____

_____

The Changes I Can Feel: _____

_____

_____

_____

_____

_____

_____

_____

_____

16
WEEK

Quote of the Week

The greatest thing about man is his ability to transcend himself, his ancestry, and his environment and to become what he dreams of being.

—Tully C. Knoles

THIS WEEK'S MENTAL TIP

You were born a blank slate when it comes to writing any dream in your heart and making it real in your life. You are an unlimited source of imagination and power when it comes to creating the life you want. And if you aren't living that dream life of yours, one of the biggest reasons is because you won't allow yourself to live it. You see, nowhere is it written that your life should or must fit the mold or expectations of what you think your family, friends or society expects from you. They were given their lives to do with them as they choose, and you were given your life to be whoever and do whatever you choose. If your life was meant for others to decide, it would've been given to them and not you, so break free from the lies that have held you back. Change your body. Change your life. Travel the world. Be a painter or poet. Raise a family if you want. Be anything and everything you dream, and start it today. Nothing and no one can hold you back. You have the power... today.

THIS WEEK'S EXERCISE TIP

Looking for a sure cure for the "I'm in a rut" blues? It's called the *30-Day Push,* and it can transform your body. Because your body quickly habituates (translation: *gets used to doing the same thing*), often times you'll need to not only do something completely different, but do it in unconventional ways. If you've been working out doing the same kinds of exercises, with the same weight and reps, then what your body could use is something completely different. Try doing 50% fewer sets and 50% fewer exercises, but double your workout intensity. That is, spend less time working out but lift heavier weights (only after a good warm-up) during the workout. When I say heavier, I'm not talking about an extra

5 or 10 pounds. I'm talking about using near-maximum-ability weights for fewer reps, say 3-6 reps instead of 10-12. Be prepared to be a bit sore after each workout, but the soreness will quickly go away as your body breaks out of the rut and changes by making you stronger and firmer in areas you may have thought could not change. The key is to use this type of training and any other different types you'd like to try for the next 30 days and then you can go back to a maintenance program like you were on before you started the 30-Day Push. You may find that doing the 30-Day Push every 4 months may be just the ticket to keep you progressing for years and years to come.

THIS WEEK'S NUTRITION TIP

When buying breads and grain foods, choose those that say "whole grain" on the label. Why? First, it isn't overly processed and it still has all its natural ingredients; and second, whole grains have higher fiber, which is good for that beautiful bod of yours.

16

The Little Things I Did This Week To Help Me Reach My Goal and Change My Body and Life

For Nutrition: _____

_____

_____

_____

_____

_____

_____

_____

For Exercise: _____

_____

_____

_____

_____

_____

_____

_____

_____

The Little Things I Did This Week
To Help Me Reach My Goal and
Change My Body and Life

16

For Thinking Differently: _____

_____

_____

_____

_____

_____

_____

_____

To Help Inspire Myself: _____

_____

_____

_____

_____

_____

_____

_____

_____

16

The Little Things I Did This Week To Help Me Reach My Goal and Change My Body and Life

The Changes I Can See: _____

_____

_____

_____

_____

_____

_____

_____

_____

The Changes I Can Feel: _____

_____

_____

_____

_____

_____

_____

_____

_____

17

WEEK

Quote of the Week

At every crossing on the road that leads to the future, each progressive spirit is opposed by a thousand appointed to guard the past.

—Maurice Maeterlinck

THIS WEEK'S MENTAL TIP

You can bet that for any man or woman who desired a new kind of life, there was always someone who challenged them. Even when it comes to something so simple and positive as eating just a little bit healthier and doing just a little bit more exercise to change how they look and feel, other people will bring up many reasons why you cannot or should not do it. "Remember when you tried exercising or that diet before? Look what happened," one so-called friend might quickly remind you. And remember the reactions of all those people when you told them about moving or changing jobs? The fact is, most people are so afraid of changing any part of their lives that when people with enough belief in themselves come along and want to change theirs, they are met with an army of disapproving looks, frowning faces and words meant to deflate. If you've got the desire to change, then keep that head of yours looking forward and ahead, and care not what anyone else says or thinks. Your body and your life are about to become something extraordinary.

THIS WEEK'S EXERCISE TIP

Here's something you can do anywhere, anytime, and it will give you a potent little mini-workout without going to the gym or touching a weight. I call it *tense & relax*, and it works like this: pick any muscle, let's say the biceps. Flex that arm until you feel the biceps contracting and tensing. Hold the biceps in that tensed position for anywhere from 4-10 seconds. Really tense it as hard as you can for the entire 4-10 seconds. Let that arm relax and do the same thing for the other arm. For the chest, put both arms straight out in front of you and don't allow them to touch as you squeeze the chest together. For triceps, simply let the arm hang down to your side and tense the triceps as you straighten the arm. The trick is to keep the maximum amount of tension—for those 4-10 seconds—on the muscle you want to work. The harder the contraction, the better the result.

THIS WEEK'S NUTRITION TIP

Almost everyone loves chocolate, but no one loves the high calories it has. And with more news coming out about the health benefits of eating "moderate" amounts of chocolate every so often, is there a way you can have that chocolate and feel good about it too? You bet. Whenever possible, try using unsweetened cocoa powder in those recipes, since cocoa powder is chocolate, but with most of the fat removed.

17

The Little Things I Did This Week To Help Me Reach My Goal and Change My Body and Life

For Nutrition: _____

_____

_____

_____

_____

_____

_____

_____

For Exercise: _____

_____

_____

_____

_____

_____

_____

_____

The Little Things I Did This Week To Help Me Reach My Goal and Change My Body and Life

17

For Thinking Differently: _____

_____

_____

_____

_____

_____

_____

_____

To Help Inspire Myself: _____

_____

_____

_____

_____

_____

_____

_____

17

The Little Things I Did This Week To Help Me Reach My Goal and Change My Body and Life

The Changes I Can See:

_____

_____

_____

_____

_____

_____

_____

_____

The Changes I Can Feel:

_____

_____

_____

_____

_____

_____

_____

_____

18
WEEK

Quote of the Week

The vision of things to be done may come a long time before the way of doing them becomes clear, but woe to him that distrusts the vision.

—Jenkin Lloyd Jones

THIS WEEK'S MENTAL TIP

Each day you awake, you will be faced with different challenges, new and old problems to solve, actions and events to understand and lessons to learn. Many times, it may all seem totally overwhelming. Just relax, for it's completely natural and just another day in the University of Life where class never ends. And in the midst of everything that happens in your life, you may be confused, since it seems like you'll have no idea of what to do next or how things will turn out. And in your seemingly endless search for the right answer, you may get a feeling, an intuitive hunch—often when you least expect it—of what feels like the right thing to do. This feeling may come and go quickly, before you go back to doing what you've always done; and that is, to keep thinking and thinking about the problem and worrying yourself into an unhappy and uneasy state of mind. But let's go back to that hunch. More times than not, that hunch is the right answer and direction for you to follow. It comes deep inside your mind—away from the daily distractions—and it's giving you the right direction and action you must take to solve that problem or understand that situation and life lesson. Listen to that hunch and follow it, wherever or however strange it may seem. You may not have all the answers on know the roads it will take you down when you begin. But if you trust Life and the vision and inner "knowing" you feel, you are sure to be led to the right road, with the right people and events that will help you, all at the right time.

THIS WEEK'S EXERCISE TIP

People love snow skiing, and I'm going to give you a terrific workout that you can do while skiing. No need to ski fast or do tough moguls for this one. Simply changing leg positions is all that's needed for an amazing leg workout. Start out by keeping your knees slightly bent as you ski. After a few hundred feet, bend your legs even more, lowering your body just a few inches lower than when you started. Hold your legs in this position for at least 2-3 minutes, and then return your legs to the starting position. The more your legs approach the straight up-and-down position, the less resistance and easier it is. However, the more you bend your legs and lower your body, the harder it will be. Do combinations of low resistance with minimal leg bend to high resistance with lots of leg bend for a day on the slopes your legs and body will not soon forget.

THIS WEEK'S NUTRITION TIP

If you're hankerin' for a good, old-fashioned hot dog, go for the low-fat and nonfat turkey or chicken franks. I know, you're thinking a hot dog should be beef or pork, but take a good look at the label next time you're in the store. Some of those regular hot dogs can have upwards of 15 grams of fat *per* frank.

18

The Little Things I Did This Week
To Help Me Reach My Goal and
Change My Body and Life

For Nutrition: _____

_____

_____

_____

_____

_____

_____

_____

For Exercise: _____

_____

_____

_____

_____

_____

_____

_____

The Little Things I Did This Week
To Help Me Reach My Goal and
Change My Body and Life

18

For Thinking Differently: _____

_____

_____

_____

_____

_____

_____

_____

To Help Inspire Myself: _____

_____

_____

_____

_____

_____

_____

_____

_____

18

The Little Things I Did This Week
To Help Me Reach My Goal and
Change My Body and Life

The Changes I Can See: _____

_____

_____

_____

_____

_____

_____

_____

The Changes I Can Feel: _____

_____

_____

_____

_____

_____

_____

_____

_____

19
WEEK

Quote of the Week

Careful is the person who pauses before changing their lives or making their plans based on the promises of others.

THIS WEEK'S MENTAL TIP

Others mean well. They tell us things, promise us things and want to give us things, but many times they don't come through. After all, they experience the same thing from other people too, so who can blame them for things they cannot control? It's almost like an endless chain connecting people and events in the movie of life. When it happens to others, it's easy to chalk it up as "human nature," except when it becomes your happiness that depends on other people's promises and actions. Take having a workout partner. You promise each other that you'll exercise together or start that new diet together. So you get yourself all happy and excited and, lo and behold, that day comes when they cannot meet you or forget to meet you for a workout. Even though they've promised, life happens and plans and people change. Just understand it for what it is and let it go. You've learned a powerful lesson: When it comes to changing or experiencing anything in your life, the only one you can depend on 100% of the time is *you*. If others want to share in those experiences, then great. But with or without anyone else, simply live your life, look and feel the way you want, and depend on yourself, and you won't be disappointed.

THIS WEEK'S EXERCISE TIP

If you love the water and are looking for an awesome cross-training workout, then rowing is your answer. Besides cross-country skiing in the winter, rowing ranks right near the top for one of the most effective aerobic and resistance exercises you can do. Here are a few things to keep in mind to get great results from it. Number one: Big, long and sweeping strokes demand more brief and intense bursts of strength to overcome the added resistance of the rowing movement.

This is a good way to take care of the resistance part of the workout. Number two: Short and quick strokes, while they may not require the quick power surges needed to move the paddles through the larger amounts of water and distance, do require more endurance for the increased number of strokes in order to move you and the boat over the same distance. This is a great way to train for the aerobic/cardio portion of your workout. When you combine both, you get a marvelous way to condition your body.

THIS WEEK'S NUTRITION TIP

Many people are confused when they hear they should be eating a certain number of servings of this or that food or from a food group. So, do you know how big a serving is? Here's an easy way: ½ to 1 cup of cooked or raw vegetables is one serving, ½ cup of vegetable or fruit juice is one serving and one medium size piece of fruit is also one serving. And what about food portion sizes for fish, fowl or meat? Go for a serving of about 3-4 ounces—that's about the size of a computer mouse or folded wallet.

19

The Little Things I Did This Week To Help Me Reach My Goal and Change My Body and Life

For Nutrition: _____

_____

_____

_____

_____

_____

_____

_____

_____

For Exercise: _____

_____

_____

_____

_____

_____

_____

_____

_____

The Little Things I Did This Week To Help Me Reach My Goal and Change My Body and Life

19

For Thinking Differently:

_____

_____

_____

_____

_____

_____

_____

To Help Inspire Myself:

_____

_____

_____

_____

_____

_____

_____

19

The Little Things I Did This Week To Help Me Reach My Goal and Change My Body and Life

The Changes I Can See: _____

_____

_____

_____

_____

_____

_____

_____

The Changes I Can Feel: _____

_____

_____

_____

_____

_____

_____

_____

_____

20
WEEK

Quote of the Week

My mother said to me, "If you become a soldier you'll be a general; if you become a monk you'll end up as the pope." Instead, I became a painter and wound up as Picasso.

—Pablo Picasso

THIS WEEK'S MENTAL TIP

If we all had parents like Picasso's mother, who filled us with such love and belief, what a changed world we'd have. As I read that quote again, it says to me, if you follow the calling of your life and use the desires you have and the talents inside you, then you can become a Picasso in whatever career or life calling you have. The point is to follow those desires and dreams and allow them to fill your life to overflowing with the incredible abundance of experiences and rewards that are waiting for you right now. No matter who you are, where you live, how young or old, how short or tall, or what religion, color or creed, you are a Picasso right now; a living masterpiece that Life has created for you and the world to enjoy. Simply follow your heart and dreams wherever they lead you; by doing so, you'll bless the world and it will pour its blessings upon you.

THIS WEEK'S EXERCISE TIP

As they say, human nature tends to be more on the lazy side. So, if you're looking for a novel way to get a light, little workout, look no further than your refrigerator. But you're going to need two one-gallon plastic jugs of juice, milk or water. Hold each of those gallon jugs in your hands and think of them as if they were dumbbells in the gym. Give yourself a quickie arm pump by doing a fast set of 25 reps. How about raising and lowering the jugs out to your sides for 12 reps for a nice little delt (shoulder) pump? Do this either early in the morning before breakfast or before dinner, and you may find that, while this may not radically change your body, it will get the blood pumping; and many times, that's enough to release those powerful exercise-produced endorphins that de-stress you and invigorate mind and body.

116

THIS WEEK'S NUTRITION TIP

Did you know that a 4-ounce serving of french fries has almost three times the calories and more than 10 times the waist-expanding amount of fat when compared to the same sized 4-ounce baked potato? If you love french fries (and who doesn't?), then instead of frying, try baking them for great taste with minimal fat.

20

The Little Things I Did This Week To Help Me Reach My Goal and Change My Body and Life

For Nutrition: _____

_____

_____

_____

_____

_____

_____

_____

For Exercise: _____

_____

_____

_____

_____

_____

_____

_____

The Little Things I Did This Week
To Help Me Reach My Goal and
Change My Body and Life

20

For Thinking Differently: _____

_____

_____

_____

_____

_____

_____

To Help Inspire Myself: _____

_____

_____

_____

_____

_____

_____

_____

20

The Little Things I Did This Week To Help Me Reach My Goal and Change My Body and Life

The Changes I Can See:

_____

_____

_____

_____

_____

_____

_____

_____

The Changes I Can Feel:

_____

_____

_____

_____

_____

_____

_____

_____

21

WEEK

Quote of the Week

I am not interested in the past. I am interested in the future, for that is where I expect to spend the rest of my life.

—Charles F. Kettering

THIS WEEK'S MENTAL TIP

Why do you think it's so hard for people to let go of the past? And why is it so unnecessarily tough for people to let go of the false ideas and myths about their bodies? For example, a person looks and feels a certain way for a number of years, has tried numerous diets, bought lots of exercise gizmos and machines and still, they always go back to looking and feeling like their old selves. So what's wrong here? A big reason is that they still have the same old picture of how they are supposed to look floating inside their head and, along with that, the limiting beliefs about themselves that keep that picture alive, day after day, year after frustrating year. It's time we change that. From this day on, one of the most powerful things you can do to change how you look and feel is first give your brain a new picture on the inside that you want it to create on the outside. All lasting change must first come from inside before it shows up on the outside. Along with that new picture of how you want to look, think more and more each day about how great and happy you'll feel once that new picture of you actually begins to happen. You'll find yourself starting to feel good about yourself again, and it really will start to sink in that, yes, this new you is really going to happen. And believe me, it most certainly will.

THIS WEEK'S EXERCISE TIP

One exercise that's just as good today as it was when you were a kid is cycling. In gyms, they're all over the place and you may even have one at home. But the real fun of cycling is when you're doing it again outdoors. Here are a few ways to change the look of your legs simply by changing how you cycle. First, if you want thinner and leaner looking thighs, simply use higher gears when you pedal, which will create less resistance and easier, yet faster strokes. If you want a bit more muscular legs, then spend more time using the lower gears of the bike, which will create more resistance and slower strokes.

THIS WEEK'S NUTRITION TIP

Many people love carbohydrates. Granted, they're important for energy for the body. However, excess carbohydrates can be a real no-no if you want a leaner and more shapely body. Excess carbohydrates—yes, even those sweet treats that have "fat free" on the label—are stored as fat. When the body breaks down carbohydrates for its use, they eventually form pyruvic acid, and this puts a damper on how the body uses and gets rid of body fat. Eating too many carbohydrates (especially the wrong kinds of empty-calorie foods made with white sugar) can cause B-vitamin deficiency as the body uses its B vitamins in order to process the carbohydrates. The best kinds of carbohydrates to eat are fresh vegetables, fresh fruits and whole grains and cereals. Just be careful that you don't eat too many of them.

21

The Little Things I Did This Week To Help Me Reach My Goal and Change My Body and Life

For Nutrition: _____

_____

_____

_____

_____

_____

_____

_____

_____

For Exercise: _____

_____

_____

_____

_____

_____

_____

_____

_____

The Little Things I Did This Week To Help Me Reach My Goal and Change My Body and Life

21

For Thinking Differently:

_____

_____

_____

_____

_____

_____

_____

To Help Inspire Myself:

_____

_____

_____

_____

_____

_____

_____

_____

21

The Little Things I Did This Week To Help Me Reach My Goal and Change My Body and Life

The Changes I Can See: _____

_____

_____

_____

_____

_____

_____

_____

_____

The Changes I Can Feel: _____

_____

_____

_____

_____

_____

_____

_____

_____

_____

22
WEEK

Quote of the Week

If we were to do all that we are capable of doing, we would literally astonish ourselves.

—Thomas A. Edison

THIS WEEK'S MENTAL TIP

Ever thought about what you are truly capable of achieving and doing? I'm not talking about what you have done in the past or are now doing. I'm talking about your untapped potential. Society and most family and friends are so used to doing only just enough—little more—at their jobs, at school, in relationships or in anything else to keep things going smoothly. After all, they reason, why do more if you don't need to? And that's the rub. Little do they know that only a *little more* knowledge, a *little more* belief or a *little more* effort is often the biggest thing that separates someone who rises to the top from the majority who settle for crumbs and doing less than their best. Here's a wee bit of change-your-life advice: Do just a *little bit more* than you're doing now, in any area of your life, and the results just might astonish you. The difference between the racehorse that wins the big prize and the second place finisher that doesn't is often only a split second.

THIS WEEK'S EXERCISE TIP

Ever dream you could get in better shape each time you shop? That's got to be the best of both worlds. A very simple way to get your heart pumping, blood flowing and muscles working is by increasing the distance of walking you'd normally do during any given day. When you arrive at the mall, office, restaurant, theater, school or anywhere you go, simply park the car farther away. Next, when leaving wherever you go, try using the opposite entrance you came in. The extra distance can make a big difference. Finally, when given a choice of stairs or the escalator, always use the stairs.

THIS WEEK'S NUTRITION TIP

You know a good diet helps keep you healthy and a bad diet does just the opposite. You also have a good idea, without reading book after book or seeing a nutritional guru, which foods are good for your body and which ones make it sluggish. What you may not know is which kinds of foods give your body the extra power of antioxidants (those little warriors that help keep your body healthy). Here are a few to eat more of:

1. Fresh fruits and vegetables are best—and the darker the colors the more better—and next on the list would be the frozen varieties.

2. Go for the fruits over the juices.

3. Pick red grapes over white ones.

4. Eat more raw vegetables like broccoli and cauliflower.

5. When cooking, use extra virgin olive oil.

6. Eat more yellow or red onions.

7. Choose pink grapefruit and not white.

22

The Little Things I Did This Week To Help Me Reach My Goal and Change My Body and Life

For Nutrition: _____

_____

_____

_____

_____

_____

_____

_____

For Exercise: _____

_____

_____

_____

_____

_____

_____

_____

The Little Things I Did This Week
To Help Me Reach My Goal and
Change My Body and Life

22

For Thinking Differently: _____

_____

_____

_____

_____

_____

_____

_____

To Help Inspire Myself: _____

_____

_____

_____

_____

_____

_____

_____

_____

22

The Little Things I Did This Week To Help Me Reach My Goal and Change My Body and Life

The Changes I Can See:

_____

_____

_____

_____

_____

_____

_____

_____

The Changes I Can Feel:

_____

_____

_____

_____

_____

_____

_____

_____

23
WEEK

Quote of the Week

Success is to be measured not so much by the position that one has reached in life as by the obstacles which he has overcome while trying to succeed.

—Booker T. Washington

THIS WEEK'S MENTAL TIP

Be assured that you won't achieve success in your life or change your body unless you go through some adversity on your path to get to your destination. There are no free rides in life, and thank goodness for that! Adversity, hardship, pain and discomfort are incredibly powerful forces that transform us. If you're experiencing any of them right now, then there's much to be happy about, for all those things are changing you—changing your beliefs, changing your attitudes, changing your discipline, changing your actions and changing your body and life to be something better, something more. Great workouts that build a great body come from the experiences gained from less-than-great workouts when one starts out. You overcome the obstacles and sticking points by weeding out the things that don't work, to find the things that do. Life is just the same. Always remember it.

THIS WEEK'S EXERCISE TIP

Traveling can be a real detour to even the best exercise plans. Delays, late arrivals, different foods and lack of sleep don't help when you've been on a good schedule that's bringing you good results. Yet, there are some things you can do while you're on the plane that will help. When you're flying, drink more water. Some experts say a person's body loses one pint of water for every hour they fly, due to cabin pressure and processed air. Alcohol is another big factor in dehydration, so if you're having a drink, have an equal amount of water. Eat less salty foods and snacks. Those pretzels, chips and snack mixes they give you are tasty, but they're loaded with sodium, so don't go overboard. Every 30 minutes or so, get up out of your seat and walk to the back of the plane. Sitting in a cramped seat with legs bent and being inactive doesn't do your body any favors, either. So while you're seated, do some heel lifts (i.e., calf raises) and extend those legs straight out in front of you (if you can); and every 30-45 minutes, get up and walk up or down the aisle.

THIS WEEK'S NUTRITION TIP

Go to your kitchen and grab a tablespoon, because what I 'm going to tell you to put in it will give you an amazing amount of 17 vitamins (even all those B vitamins), 14 minerals (including those trace minerals) and 16 amino acids—and it's only about 20-25 calories (depending on how much you can fit onto that spoon). I'm talking about Brewer's Yeast. You can put it on cereal, in yogurt or in cottage cheese; you can sprinkle it over any foods like salads or mix it into any of your other favorite dishes. Try one tablespoon a day for that extra iron and vitamin one-two punch.

23

The Little Things I Did This Week To Help Me Reach My Goal and Change My Body and Life

For Nutrition: _____

_____

_____

_____

_____

_____

_____

_____

_____

For Exercise: _____

_____

_____

_____

_____

_____

_____

_____

_____

The Little Things I Did This Week To Help Me Reach My Goal and Change My Body and Life

23

For Thinking Differently: _____

_____

_____

_____

_____

_____

_____

_____

To Help Inspire Myself: _____

_____

_____

_____

_____

_____

_____

_____

23

The Little Things I Did This Week To Help Me Reach My Goal and Change My Body and Life

The Changes I Can See:

_____

_____

_____

_____

_____

_____

_____

_____

The Changes I Can Feel:

_____

_____

_____

_____

_____

_____

_____

_____

24
WEEK

Quote of the Week

Nurture your mind with great thoughts, for you will never go any higher than you think.

—Benjamin Disraeli

THIS WEEK'S MENTAL TIP

"Where the mind goes, the body follows" is a maxim I've found to be 100% true. For you can only go as high as your thoughts and beliefs in yourself. And who sets the limits on those beliefs? You do. Beliefs come from our thoughts, for what we think about, we most certainly bring about. If you have the belief that you'll always be overweight, out of shape and look and feel the same, then those thoughts become your limits and you'll never go beyond those boundaries unless and until you change those thoughts to match the changes you want to see happen, the new image of how you want to look and feel.

THIS WEEK'S EXERCISE TIP

Last week, we talked about what you can do on the plane. So what do you do once you arrive at your destination? Depending on when you arrive (many international flights arrive the next morning), you'll want to stay awake during the day and make your bedtime at night, even if it's as early as 7:00 p.m. This will help keep your body clock in its regular awake/day-sleep/night mode. After checking in to your destination, and as soon as possible, either do a bit of light exercise in your hotel room or, better yet, go for a relaxing sightseeing walk around the city. Just stay active and keep moving as much as you enjoyably can. Eat light meals throughout the day, as having high-fat or high-calorie meals will only make you tired. Some people, when they do long international flights, have found melatonin (an over-the-counter supplement found in a variety of stores) to be a good way to knock off the effects of jet lag, some say, by as much as a few days. About 90 minutes or so before bedtime, you might try having a light meal with a bit more protein.

As a tired traveler, you sure don't want a hungry, growling stomach to wake you up in the middle of the night and make it difficult for you to become tired again and fall back to sleep.

THIS WEEK'S NUTRITION TIP

Occasionally you may have an upset stomach, and many of the foods you eat and drink (such as salty and fried foods, mayonnaise, fruit juices, coffee and meat) can be likely culprits. For years, people have believed eating a banana a day helps calm the queezies, so you might want to give that a try. Others swear by tea. Another great natural way to soothe an upset stomach or even motion sickness is by taking ginger. Now you know why Grandma and Mom gave you a little ginger ale when you had that upset tummy.

24

The Little Things I Did This Week To Help Me Reach My Goal and Change My Body and Life

For Nutrition: _____

_____

_____

_____

_____

_____

_____

_____

_____

For Exercise: _____

_____

_____

_____

_____

_____

_____

_____

_____

The Little Things I Did This Week
To Help Me Reach My Goal and
Change My Body and Life

24

For Thinking Differently: _____

_____

_____

_____

_____

_____

_____

_____

To Help Inspire Myself: _____

_____

_____

_____

_____

_____

_____

_____

24

The Little Things I Did This Week To Help Me Reach My Goal and Change My Body and Life

The Changes I Can See: _____

_____

_____

_____

_____

_____

_____

_____

_____

The Changes I Can Feel: _____

_____

_____

_____

_____

_____

_____

_____

_____

25
WEEK

Quote of the Week

*I am an old man and have known a great many
troubles, but most of them never happened.*

—Mark Twain

THIS WEEK'S MENTAL TIP

A very wise person once said, "The majority of things in life we worry about never happen and the very few things that do, are 9 times out of 10, either beyond our control or they're not as bad as they seem." So what have you been worrying about? And, more to the point, why? Life's much too short to waste time thinking about things that most likely will never happen.

THIS WEEK'S EXERCISE TIP

Remember those big beach or gym balls you used to hit around when you were a kid? Well, they've made a comeback and are excellent at toning abs and lower back. You'll want to use one that's at least 2-3 feet in diameter. Place the ball on the floor and center the middle of your back over it. Keep your glutes against the ball and your legs spread apart about 1-2 feet. Keep your feet firmly planted on the floor, and keep the feet about 2-3 feet apart. Cross your arms across your chest and keep your head up. Slowly raise your upper body forward towards your legs for a few inches, hold it there for 1-2 seconds and then slowly lower it back down again; then begin again, without stopping at the bottom of the exercise. Do at least 15-25 reps.

THIS WEEK'S NUTRITION TIP

Here's a little trick you can use to fool your brain into thinking you've eaten more than you actually have, and it can work great for dropping those extra fat pounds. Try using smaller plates and utensils. Not only will it reduce the amount of food you can put on them at any given time, you'll have to take more bites just to get the same portions you would if you used those big spoons, forks and plates. Along with that, try eating slower. Many times, we eat so fast that we keep eating when our bodies are already full, yet the signal from the stomach to the brain hasn't had enough time to catch up and tell us to stop. When eating, think slow and small, and you will be rewarded.

25

The Little Things I Did This Week To Help Me Reach My Goal and Change My Body and Life

For Nutrition: _____

_____

_____

_____

_____

_____

_____

_____

For Exercise: _____

_____

_____

_____

_____

_____

_____

_____

The Little Things I Did This Week
To Help Me Reach My Goal and
Change My Body and Life

For Thinking Differently:

_____

_____

_____

_____

_____

_____

_____

_____

To Help Inspire Myself:

_____

_____

_____

_____

_____

_____

_____

_____

25

The Little Things I Did This Week
To Help Me Reach My Goal and
Change My Body and Life

The Changes I Can See:

_____

_____

_____

_____

_____

_____

_____

_____

The Changes I Can Feel:

_____

_____

_____

_____

_____

_____

_____

_____

26
WEEK

Quote of the Week

If you wait for the perfect moment when all is safe and assured, it may never arrive. Mountains will not be climbed, races won, or lasting happiness achieved.

—Maurice Chevalier

THIS WEEK'S MENTAL TIP

I've got some news for you today. There will never be a more perfect time to change your body and your life than right now. There will not be a time when you'll have all the answers before you start. There will not be a time when you'll know all the uncertainties and difficulties that await you. And there will not be a time when you'll know all the happiness and rewards that await you on the way to dream and when you arrive. All you have is *today, right now, this moment*. Think of the tragedy of September 11 in New York City and all those thousands of people who perished who may have been looking forward to changing their lives or making new changes or trying new things starting the next day. Yet in seconds, it was over—no tomorrows. We don't know what's going to happen in the next hour, let alone the next day or the next year. *Right now* is yours, and it's all you've got. Grab it and make it exactly what you want.

THIS WEEK'S EXERCISE TIP

This week, we're still having a ball (as in exercise ball), and I'll tell you how to use to strengthen your lower back. Using the same size ball as I told you about last week, place the front of your body over the ball. Be sure only the stomach and upper thighs touch the ball. You don't want to have the ball touching the chest or neck. Spread your legs out wide—about 2-4 feet—and keep your toes touching the floor at all times. Clasp your hands and place them and your arms behind your head. Slowly raise your upper body up from the ball for a few inches, hold it there for 1-2 seconds, then slowly lower it back down and begin again. Be sure to not over-extend the upper body by raising it too far up or too fast. Slow, steady and controlled movement is what you want. Do three sets of 5-9 reps once a week.

THIS WEEK'S NUTRITION TIP

If you love being active and want to eat foods that will be good for those joints, then start eating more fish foods high in omega-3 fatty acids such as salmon, mackerel, trout and sardines.

26

The Little Things I Did This Week To Help Me Reach My Goal and Change My Body and Life

For Nutrition: _____

_____

_____

_____

_____

_____

_____

_____

For Exercise: _____

_____

_____

_____

_____

_____

_____

_____

The Little Things I Did This Week To Help Me Reach My Goal and Change My Body and Life

26

For Thinking Differently:

_____

_____

_____

_____

_____

_____

_____

_____

To Help Inspire Myself:

_____

_____

_____

_____

_____

_____

_____

_____

26

The Little Things I Did This Week To Help Me Reach My Goal and Change My Body and Life

The Changes I Can See: _____

_____

_____

_____

_____

_____

_____

_____

_____

The Changes I Can Feel: _____

_____

_____

_____

_____

_____

_____

_____

_____

27
WEEK

Quote of the Week

I love you for what you are, but I love you yet more for what you are going to be.

I love you not so much for your realities as for your ideals. I pray for your desires that they may be great, rather than for your satisfactions, which may be so hazardously little.

—Charles Sandburg

THIS WEEK'S MENTAL TIP

On the one hand, you have those who say much of our problem as men and women comes from our not being satisfied in what we have and our always wanting more. On the other hand, you have those who say our problem lies in the opposite: settling for less than we are capable of. So who's right? Are any of them? A good rule of thumb I've found is a simple test: If you look outside yourself for happiness and validation in people and material things, then happiness and fulfillment will elude you; If you are essentially a happy person with or without the accolades of worldly success or the need to possess and acquire things, then the need to grow, expand, become and experience comes from a knowing deep inside you, that as you grow, you are capable of much more. And it'll be the same when you reach your dream and goal of a new looking and feeling body. It's only human to think, before you have it, that once you get it that'll be all you'll need or want. But once you reach your goal of a changed body and a changed you, which you most certainly will, then a brand new road and vista opens up to you—one you never could have imagined when you started—from which new goals and dreams can begin. This is the beautiful dance of life, and one you'll deeply enjoy. Just be sure your head and heart are in the right place, and you'll have a lifetime of enjoyment.

THIS WEEK'S EXERCISE TIP

Using the stairs can be a great way to get a workout. One way is to do lunges. Lunges are a terrific leg exercise and will work wonders to shape, tone and strengthen your thighs. Begin by placing one leg on the first step and the other leg in line under your upper body. Look forward, keep the upper body erect and allow the leg under your body to bend. Start off by lowering the body for a few inches, then back up to the starting position. After a few reps, lower the knee of the leg that's under your body, until your knee is only a few inches above the floor. Do 10-20 reps for each leg. To make it a tougher workout, put your frontmost leg on the second or third stair; the farther the distance between the non-stair/non-working leg and the other leg, the more difficult the exercise becomes.

THIS WEEK'S NUTRITION TIP

You work hard at school, your career, raising your family, enjoying life and staying fit and healthy, but for many people the sight of varicose veins in the legs doesn't bring a smile. So can you do anything to help prevent or minimize those pesky looking things? First, check to be sure you're getting enough vitamin E in your diet, since vitamin E acts as a blood vessel dilator and helps keep circulation moving freely and smoothly. And when it's time to relax, give that body a rest and don't relax sitting up. Lie down and elevate your feet so they are slightly higher than your head.

27

The Little Things I Did This Week To Help Me Reach My Goal and Change My Body and Life

For Nutrition: _____

_____

_____

_____

_____

_____

_____

_____

For Exercise: _____

_____

_____

_____

_____

_____

_____

_____

The Little Things I Did This Week
To Help Me Reach My Goal and
Change My Body and Life

27

For Thinking Differently: _____

_____

_____

_____

_____

_____

_____

To Help Inspire Myself: _____

_____

_____

_____

_____

_____

_____

_____

27

The Little Things I Did This Week
To Help Me Reach My Goal and
Change My Body and Life

The Changes I Can See:

_____

_____

_____

_____

_____

_____

_____

_____

The Changes I Can Feel:

_____

_____

_____

_____

_____

_____

_____

_____

28
WEEK

Quote of the Week

Ideals are like stars: you will not succeed in touching them with your hands, but like the seafaring man on the ocean desert of waters, you choose them as your guides, and following them, you reach your destiny.

—Carl Schurz

THIS WEEK'S MENTAL TIP

I can tell you with absolute certainty that the path you think you'll be taking when you begin your journey to change your body and life will turn out to be amazingly different once you reach that goal. Look back at what has happened in your life and where you were just 12 months ago, and look at where you are and who you are today. Talk about changes! And the same is going to happen to you when you begin exercising and being more active again or getting back to eating more healthy and treating your body better. Always keep in mind the goal and dream and keep looking up to those as your guides, like stars in the sky at night, as you begin traveling down your new road to your dream. But always know that the road you take will not be a straight one; it will have many hills, bumps, curves, potholes and twists before you reach that point, just over the horizon, when you arrive at the destination of a new you and a new life.

THIS WEEK'S EXERCISE TIP

We're not finished *stairing* yet. Here are a few other ways to make the stairs your gym away from the gym. First, when walking up the stairs, try taking two or three stairs at a time instead of the usual one. Next, try going up the stairs sideways and backwards. You'll feel this work the leg muscles differently. To increase endurance and aerobic benefits, try brisk walking up and down the stairs. When that becomes easy, start doing a slow run up the stairs, followed by a regular walk down them. To get an even better workout, you can increase the speed of your walk or run up the stairs, run up a greater number of stairs, or do fewer stairs but do them faster and more times.

THIS WEEK'S NUTRITION TIP

If you're taking calcium and iron supplements, don't take them at the same time. Taking them at the same time causes an interaction, which in turn causes the body to not absorb the iron. Drinks such as coffee and tea also get in the way of absorption. However, juices like orange or tomato help the body absorb that iron. Try taking the iron supplement with your meal or with tomato and orange juice and then take the calcium supplement 60–90 minutes later.

28

The Little Things I Did This Week To Help Me Reach My Goal and Change My Body and Life

For Nutrition: _____

_____

_____

_____

_____

_____

_____

_____

For Exercise: _____

_____

_____

_____

_____

_____

_____

_____

The Little Things I Did This Week
To Help Me Reach My Goal and
Change My Body and Life

28

For Thinking Differently: _____

_____

_____

_____

_____

_____

_____

_____

To Help Inspire Myself: _____

_____

_____

_____

_____

_____

_____

_____

_____

28

The Little Things I Did This Week To Help Me Reach My Goal and Change My Body and Life

The Changes I Can See: _____

_____

_____

_____

_____

_____

_____

_____

The Changes I Can Feel: _____

_____

_____

_____

_____

_____

_____

_____

_____

29
WEEK

Quote of the Week

No man ever became great or good except through many and great mistakes.

—William E. Gladstone

THIS WEEK'S MENTAL TIP

When I began working out, in my unbridled passion for the possible I made about every mistake there was to make. I worked out too hard, I worked out too much and too often, I listened to everyone but myself as to what was the best exercise program for me and I held other people's opinions higher than my own and gave them more credit than they deserved for knowing better than me how to change my body and life. Yet it was through those mistakes that I began getting frustrated, not only with my lack of progress, but also with not following my instincts of knowing what I needed to do, when and how I needed to do it and then just doing it. Once I realized my mistakes, I quickly changed my actions, listened to myself and followed my own road, and the results and success I realized have been wonderful. Never fear making mistakes. Rather, I'd say, fear not making *any*.

THIS WEEK'S EXERCISE TIP

If you've been looking for a great way to shape, firm and tone those outer thighs, at home and without any equipment, then this is for you. They're side leg raises, and you do them three ways. *First,* with knees bent. Stand up straight and hold onto either the wall, doorknob or stair rail for balance and support. With the right leg bent at the knee and foot on the floor, bend the left knee so your left foot is behind you and the leg you are about to lift is in an L-shape (upper leg straight up and down and calf and foot extended behind you). Keep the left upper leg in a straight line with your body. Raise that left leg up and out to your side as high as you can. Hold it at the top for 1-2 seconds, then slowly bring the leg back down and repeat. Do it for 15 reps, then do the same thing for the other leg. *The next way* you'll do these is by having the leg with the elevated knee not all the way bent, but at approximately ¾ extension; That is, slightly bent and not fully extended. Do the same exercise for the same number of reps. *Last but not least,* do the exercise with no bend in the knees but with legs straight and locked. You'll find this last way to be the most difficult of all, and you may not be able to lift your leg as high as you did doing it the other two ways, but that's okay. Just raise it up and out to your side as high as you can and keep those reps going until finished.

THIS WEEK'S NUTRITION TIP

You've heard for years how people swear by vitamin C as a cheap way to get over a cold. But did you know a little supplement you can buy at your health food store called zinc gluconate with glycine may also do the trick? A Dartmouth University study showed this supplement knocks out a cold over 40% faster than vitamin C.

29

The Little Things I Did This Week To Help Me Reach My Goal and Change My Body and Life

For Nutrition: _____

_____

_____

_____

_____

_____

_____

_____

_____

For Exercise: _____

_____

_____

_____

_____

_____

_____

_____

_____

The Little Things I Did This Week
To Help Me Reach My Goal and
Change My Body and Life

29

For Thinking Differently:

_____
_____
_____
_____
_____
_____
_____
_____

To Help Inspire Myself:

_____
_____
_____
_____
_____
_____
_____
_____

29

The Little Things I Did This Week
To Help Me Reach My Goal and
Change My Body and Life

The Changes I Can See: _____

_____

_____

_____

_____

_____

_____

_____

The Changes I Can Feel: _____

_____

_____

_____

_____

_____

_____

_____

30
WEEK

Quote of the Week

Cease to inquire what the future has in store, and take as a gift whatever the day brings forth.

—Horace

THIS WEEK'S MENTAL TIP

Today you may have a great workout and eat the ideal foods, and yet tomorrow your workout and diet may be the pits. But that's life and it's totally okay. Some days, we are happier than others, and things in our life just click like magic. Other days, we can do the same things in the same ways and hardly anything seems to happen. Instead of letting those not-so-good days get the best of you, go ahead and let them go and realize on that day, it'll be a day you'll take the pressure off yourself and your expectations and you'll just do the best you can, regardless of the results. Enjoy either working out or not working out; either eating healthy or not eating healthy; or anything else that comes your way. Just be happy and grateful for another precious and priceless day in that life of yours.

THIS WEEK'S EXERCISE TIP

What would you think if you could get really good at whatever sport or activity you enjoy, without having to actually do it? Well, you can. I call it *shadow practice,* and the results may surprise you. Ever watch a boxer act like he/she was boxing, doing all the punches and making all the foot and body moves, without wearing any gloves or having an opponent in front of them? They were shadow practicing, and it helps them tremendously prepare for the real event. Basketball players do it too. In fact, a number of years ago a group of researchers did a study that compared one group who shot baskets each day to another who only practiced shooting baskets mentally to a third group who did nothing. The results were surprising. As you might imagine, the group that did nothing didn't improve. However, the group that simply practiced mentally shooting baskets had nearly the same results as those who actually, physically did it! So, if you want to improve your game, whatever it may be, give shadow practicing a try.

THIS WEEK'S NUTRITION TIP

You say you just ate those foods that cause cavities and don't have your mouthwash close by? No problem. Drink some tea; it's a powerful anti-cavity drink. You can also swig down milk, coffee, grape juice or black-cherry juice. As for anti-cavity foods, go for the cheeses such as Swiss, Brie, Monterey, Gouda, Cheddar, Mozzarella or Jack. But watch the fat and calories—don't eat a lot of them.

30

The Little Things I Did This Week To Help Me Reach My Goal and Change My Body and Life

For Nutrition: _____

_____

_____

_____

_____

_____

_____

_____

_____

For Exercise: _____

_____

_____

_____

_____

_____

_____

_____

_____

The Little Things I Did This Week To Help Me Reach My Goal and Change My Body and Life

30

For Thinking Differently: _____

_____

_____

_____

_____

_____

_____

_____

To Help Inspire Myself: _____

_____

_____

_____

_____

_____

_____

_____

_____

30

The Little Things I Did This Week To Help Me Reach My Goal and Change My Body and Life

The Changes I Can See:

_____

_____

_____

_____

_____

_____

_____

_____

The Changes I Can Feel:

_____

_____

_____

_____

_____

_____

_____

_____

31
WEEK

Quote of the Week

If you have been wise and successful I congratulate you; unless you are unable to forget how successful you have been, then I pity you.

—Napoleon Hill

THIS WEEK'S MENTAL TIP

Every day and for the rest of your life, always stay humble and keep learning. The ancients have a philosophy about those who do not. They are like a cup that is too full and one that quickly grows stagnant. Yet as long as the cup stays empty, fresh water can be poured into it and therefore it will never go stale.

THIS WEEK'S EXERCISE TIP

The stair stepper and elliptical trainer have to be two of the most frequently used machines in the gym. Too bad a lot of people don't do them right. How many people do you see either leaning over or holding on to the side rails (many of them with palms facing away from them) or they do these little chicken steps whereby their legs and feet are only moving a few inches up and down? All wrong. The way to get the most from using them is by placing only the balls of the feet on the foot platform, keeping the body upright without bending over, using just your fingertips to hold onto the hand rails (and only if you need support—otherwise, don't hold onto the rails at all) and taking big, full, deep steps that are all the way up and all the way down. Do it this way and then tell me if you don't "feel" the difference.

THIS WEEK'S NUTRITION TIP

Think of how many times a day you use your teeth. When you multiply that over a lifetime, it's bound to amaze you at how strong and resilient those teeth and gums are. To keep them that way for many years to come and, hopefully, for the rest of your life, brush and floss at least twice each day. Next, to keep those bones strong, be sure to get at least 1,000 mg of calcium daily (from either low-fat or nonfat yogurt, cottage cheese, skim milk, salmon or canned sardines) and keep that vitamin C intake high. That means eating red and green peppers, strawberries, oranges and other citrus fruits, broccoli or tomatoes, or taking a vitamin C supplement.

31

The Little Things I Did This Week To Help Me Reach My Goal and Change My Body and Life

For Nutrition: _____

_____

_____

_____

_____

_____

_____

_____

_____

For Exercise: _____

_____

_____

_____

_____

_____

_____

_____

_____

The Little Things I Did This Week To Help Me Reach My Goal and Change My Body and Life

31

For Thinking Differently: _____

_____

_____

_____

_____

_____

_____

_____

To Help Inspire Myself: _____

_____

_____

_____

_____

_____

_____

_____

_____

31

The Little Things I Did This Week To Help Me Reach My Goal and Change My Body and Life

The Changes I Can See: _____

_____

_____

_____

_____

_____

_____

_____

The Changes I Can Feel: _____

_____

_____

_____

_____

_____

_____

_____

32

WEEK

Quote of the Week

I cannot give you the formula for success, but I can give you the formula for failure—try to please everybody.

—Herbert Bayard Swope

THIS WEEK'S MENTAL TIP

I'd say if you're thinking of making some changes to your body and eating, then keep it to yourself and let what you do be a surprise to everyone who knows you. I cannot tell you how many times people have told me how miserable they felt after telling others what they were going to do, only to have the fires of their new goals and dreams smoldered by the cold water of negative reaction from those very people they told. The tips you are learning in this book will help you reach that new looking and feeling body, sure; but there's a good chance you'll use not only them, but others you'll discover along the way that will become "your" formula for your success. So keep the secret to yourself. I love the old saying, "Tell the world what you're going to do, but first show it."

THIS WEEK'S EXERCISE TIP

In giving you our little stair-stepper tips from last week, you didn't think I would leave out the treadmill, did you? Say no more. Many people have treadmills in their homes rather than other cardio machines, so pay attention. I'll cut to chase and tell you how to get even better results from walking on the mill. First, take long strides. Short strides don't make the muscles work like the big, long strides. Next, elevate the platform so you'll be walking on a slight-to-moderate incline. When you combine the long strides with a higher angle, you're entering "amazing results territory." Increase the speed of your walk. Walking at 3.3 mph or less really doesn't do as much to change your body as a faster gait will. Finally, don't hold onto to those side or front handrails. Swing those arms backward and forward as you walk and really put your entire body into the exercise. The more muscles you can work, the better your result.

188

THIS WEEK'S NUTRITION TIP

As you travel and dine out, when ordering, make these food words your best friends: *steamed, lean, baked, poached, grilled, roasted, fresh* and *natural*. Eat clean if you want to be lean.

32

The Little Things I Did This Week To Help Me Reach My Goal and Change My Body and Life

For Nutrition: _____

_____

_____

_____

_____

_____

_____

_____

For Exercise: _____

_____

_____

_____

_____

_____

_____

_____

The Little Things I Did This Week
To Help Me Reach My Goal and
Change My Body and Life

32

For Thinking Differently: _____

_____

_____

_____

_____

_____

_____

_____

To Help Inspire Myself: _____

_____

_____

_____

_____

_____

_____

_____

32

The Little Things I Did This Week To Help Me Reach My Goal and Change My Body and Life

The Changes I Can See:

_____

_____

_____

_____

_____

_____

_____

The Changes I Can Feel:

_____

_____

_____

_____

_____

_____

_____

33
WEEK

Quote of the Week

If people only knew how hard I worked to gain mastery, it wouldn't seem so wonderful at all.

—Michelangelo

THIS WEEK'S MENTAL TIP

Turn on the television and watch any sports star, movie star, famous singer or musician. They make what they do appear so easy that anyone can do it. And perhaps that's the deception, for the masters of their art and craft make the difficult seem simple. Yet when you read stories about their lives, you'll find that their overnight success was 20 years or more in the making; and for many, it's taken an entire lifetime of heartache, frustration, isolation, doubt, discipline, and numbing pain, to reach the pinnacle in their fields. And to think you were bummed out and thinking about quitting when you had a not-so-good workout or the diet went off track. Puts things in perspective now, doesn't it?

THIS WEEK'S EXERCISE TIP

Here's a great leg exercise (hits inner and outer thighs) you can do while sitting on the sofa watching TV, and all you'll need is a cheap little beach ball. Start off by placing the ball between your legs just above your knees. Squeeze the ball and hold it for three seconds, then relax. Do it 12 more times just like that. Next, move the ball down so it's centered between your knees. Squeeze and hold it for three seconds then do 12 more reps. Bring the ball down your legs and let it rest between your upper calves and knees. Do the same reps and 3-second squeezes. Finally, hold the ball between your ankle and calves and again do three second squeeze and hold then do 12 more reps, and you've just had a wonderful little leg workout without leaving your seat.

THIS WEEK'S NUTRITION TIP

When the cares of the world are getting the best of you and you're feeling that blood pressure begin to rise, first and foremost, stop for a moment, chill out, take 10 deep breaths and relax. Next, cut back on your sodium intake, especially from those processed packaged and canned foods. Drop a few pounds, cut back on the beer, keep doing the exercises in this book and eat more potassium and magnesium from such magnesium-rich foods as lima beans, nuts, peas, seafood and spinach, and from such potassium-rich foods as cabbage, broccoli, spinach, bananas, potatoes, corn and even orange juice.

33

The Little Things I Did This Week To Help Me Reach My Goal and Change My Body and Life

For Nutrition: _____

_____

_____

_____

_____

_____

_____

_____

For Exercise: _____

_____

_____

_____

_____

_____

_____

_____

The Little Things I Did This Week To Help Me Reach My Goal and Change My Body and Life

33

For Thinking Differently: _____

_____

_____

_____

_____

_____

_____

_____

To Help Inspire Myself: _____

_____

_____

_____

_____

_____

_____

_____

33

The Little Things I Did This Week To Help Me Reach My Goal and Change My Body and Life

The Changes I Can See: _____

_____

_____

_____

_____

_____

_____

_____

_____

The Changes I Can Feel: _____

_____

_____

_____

_____

_____

_____

_____

_____

34

WEEK

Quote of the Week

When a person finds himself, when he stops imitating and envying others, there is something in his nature that says to him, "This is it. You have found your road at last."

—Earl Nightingale

THIS WEEK'S MENTAL TIP

Fitness and glamour magazines can be a blessing or a curse: a blessing if they inspire you and give you tips and advice that will help you reach your goals; a curse if they fuel the fires of insecurity as you compare how you look to the models they feature, what you should achieve compared to what others have achieved and a sense of uncertainty for not knowing the many things they and their experts tell you. Let go of any need to compare your body and life with anything or anyone else, no matter how tempting. Keep your eyes looking forward and forget what's behind you. Look down your own road and follow your own path to your goals and dreams, and let go of the need to compare.

THIS WEEK'S EXERCISE TIP

A lot of people aren't very flexible, and as they get older and perhaps less active, this becomes even more of a problem. Here's an excellent way to limber up without even leaving home. The first stretch will have you sitting on the floor, with your back against the front of the sofa or chair. Straighten your legs out in front of you so they are in a V-position. Stretch them away from each other as far as you comfortably can, hold that position for a few seconds and then bring the legs back in and relax. Bring them back out again just a little further this time, hold that position for a few seconds and then bring the legs back in and relax. Do this for a total of 6 reps, each time trying to move the legs further apart. The next stretch will be with your feet on a wall. Simply lie on your back and put your legs up and heels on the wall in front of you. Allow the legs to spread out in that V-shape again, and do it the same way you did the feet-on-the-floor stretch. You'll find that you'll feel even more of a stretch if your body is closer to the wall and, likewise, the easier it will be the further your body is from the wall.

THIS WEEK'S NUTRITION TIP

A few nutrition tidbits from the show called *Did You Know?* Did you know...

- That diet soda, while low in calories, is high in phosphoric acid and may deplete and reduce calcium absorption by the body?

- That vitamin B complex (made up of the many B vitamins in the family) can help prevent fatigue, headache, anxiety, insomnia, loss of memory and irritability?

- That lecithin helps emulsify cholesterol and remove it from blood vessel walls, along with helping digestion and keeping nerves healthy?

- That garlic may reduce high blood pressure, lower cholesterol, raise HDL (the good cholesterol) and lower LDL (the bad cholesterol)?

- That chromium works with insulin to help metabolize sugar and may help reduce heart disease? Good sources of chromium are to be found in blackstrap molasses, whole wheat flour and brown sugar.

34

The Little Things I Did This Week
To Help Me Reach My Goal and
Change My Body and Life

For Nutrition: _____

_____

_____

_____

_____

_____

_____

_____

_____

For Exercise: _____

_____

_____

_____

_____

_____

_____

_____

_____

The Little Things I Did This Week To Help Me Reach My Goal and Change My Body and Life

34

For Thinking Differently: _____

_____

_____

_____

_____

_____

_____

_____

To Help Inspire Myself: _____

_____

_____

_____

_____

_____

_____

34

The Little Things I Did This Week To Help Me Reach My Goal and Change My Body and Life

The Changes I Can See: _____

_____

_____

_____

_____

_____

_____

_____

The Changes I Can Feel: _____

_____

_____

_____

_____

_____

_____

_____

35
WEEK

Quote of the Week

There is a time in every man's education when he arrives at the conviction that envy is ignorance, that imitation is suicide, that he must take himself for better or worse as his portion; that though the wide universe is full of good, no kernel of nourishing corn can come to him but through the toil bestowed on that plot of ground which is given him to till. The power which resides in him is new in nature, and none but he knows what that is which he can do, nor does he know until he has tried…. Trust thyself: Every heart vibrates to that iron string.

—Ralph Waldo Emerson

THIS WEEK'S MENTAL TIP

I can give you lots of tips and advice about motivation and exercise, things I know can work wonders for you, but until you trust in yourself to go ahead and give what I tell you a try, and more importantly, do what you know is right for you, then nothing is going to happen to your body or life except the same old thing. For thousands of years, the wisest people have counseled to "trust thyself." Don't look to others to give you their approval for anything you want to do with your life. If you want to be thinner, then go ahead; eat better and exercise more. If you want to change jobs or go back to school, then do it. Once you finally let go of the need of pleasing others before you please yourself, then you are on the road to freedom and of finally trusting the most important person you will ever know... *you*.

THIS WEEK'S EXERCISE TIP

One of the quickest and most simple things you can do anywhere at anytime to change your mood and physiology is deep breathing. Most people are shallow breathers, whereby they only move their body cavity minimally each time they breathe. Yet, it's when you start deep breathing that the good stuff happens inside of you. First, more oxygen intake oxygenates the blood and helps to increase blood flow. That's a good thing. Second, more oxygen to the body and brain awakens the body and immediately changes mood. It's also the technique world class athletes use to get them ready for their performance. Try this: Next time you're feeling tired, listless or a bit down in the dumps, stand up straight and take 10 big breaths in and out, and see if that doesn't surprise you.

THIS WEEK'S NUTRITION TIP

Whatever you do in your life, just remember that nothing that has happened, is happening or will happen to you is important enough to be stressed out over it. I know it may sound easier for me to say than it may be for you to do, but remember: Too much stress not only affects you not only mentally and spiritually, but also physically and nutritionally. Too much stress can cause your body to limit (and even in some cases, stop) making the hydrochloric acid (HCl) it needs to digest the foods you eat. And when that happens, proteins aren't used efficiently, which can cause allergies, bloating and gas. No need to reach for the Tums. Just turn down the mental pressure volume knob inside you and start enjoying your meals and your life again.

35

The Little Things I Did This Week To Help Me Reach My Goal and Change My Body and Life

For Nutrition: _____

_____

_____

_____

_____

_____

_____

_____

_____

For Exercise: _____

_____

_____

_____

_____

_____

_____

_____

_____

The Little Things I Did This Week To Help Me Reach My Goal and Change My Body and Life

35

For Thinking Differently: _____

_____

_____

_____

_____

_____

_____

_____

To Help Inspire Myself: _____

_____

_____

_____

_____

_____

_____

_____

35

The Little Things I Did This Week To Help Me Reach My Goal and Change My Body and Life

The Changes I Can See: _____

_____

_____

_____

_____

_____

_____

_____

_____

The Changes I Can Feel: _____

_____

_____

_____

_____

_____

_____

_____

_____

36
WEEK

Quote of the Week

What this power is, I cannot say. All I know is that it exists… and it becomes available only when you are in a state of mind in which you know exactly what you want… and are fully determined not to quit until you get it.

—Alexander Graham Bell

THIS WEEK'S MENTAL TIP

Are you ready to shake your head in amazement at what's about to happen in your life if only you'll do but one thing? Do you want to know what that one thing is? It is this: *Take action*. The world moves aside to let pass by the people who know what they want and are walking down their path toward getting it. Boldness has power in it, and obstacles in your life are demolished when you begin to take action to get that which your heart truly desires. And you *know* the difference between a little wish or a true desire that stirs something deep inside of you. That's the kind of action I'm talking about; the kind that has passionate desire behind it. And if you're at that point when enough is enough and it's finally time to make some changes in your life and maybe even change how your body looks and feels, then you've got the fire of desire, and you will have the power and will be shown the way. Open yourself up to Life's guidance and inspiration, and trust in it.

THIS WEEK'S EXERCISE TIP

Do I have something to get that butt of yours in shape—and all you have to do is sit on it! Seriously, you can do this at home, work or school; while riding in the car; or wherever you're sitting down or even standing up. I call it the *seated glute raise*. Go ahead and sit down so you'll know what it's supposed to feel like if you want to do it standing up. While seated, simply squeeze the glute muscles together and as you do, it should raise your upper body off the chair slightly. Hold it there in the elevated position for 2-3 seconds and then relax. Squeeze the muscle and feel it raise your upper body higher. The key is to really squeeze those glutes together and hold them in that position for a few seconds. Do this a few times throughout the day and do it for a good minute or so each time. No *butts* about it, you're going to like this little gem.

THIS WEEK'S NUTRITION TIP

Like frozen vegetables? Good, then I'd like to suggest a great one to always keep in your freezer. It's spinach, and it's loaded with lutein that's wonderful for your eyes, bones, brain and arteries. Oh, and Popeye likes it too!

36

The Little Things I Did This Week To Help Me Reach My Goal and Change My Body and Life

For Nutrition: _____

_____

_____

_____

_____

_____

_____

_____

For Exercise: _____

_____

_____

_____

_____

_____

_____

_____

The Little Things I Did This Week To Help Me Reach My Goal and Change My Body and Life

36

For Thinking Differently: _____

_____

_____

_____

_____

_____

_____

_____

To Help Inspire Myself: _____

_____

_____

_____

_____

_____

_____

_____

36

The Little Things I Did This Week To Help Me Reach My Goal and Change My Body and Life

The Changes I Can See: _____

_____

_____

_____

_____

_____

_____

_____

The Changes I Can Feel: _____

_____

_____

_____

_____

_____

_____

_____

37
WEEK

Quote of the Week

It is never too late to be what you might have been.

—George Eliot

THIS WEEK'S MENTAL TIP

Are you 20 years old and unsure what to do with your life? Fantastic! You say you're 30 or 40 and would like to make some changes in your life? Perfect! What? You're telling me you've hit the magic 50 or raced to 60, 70 or 80 before you even realized it? Relax... the rest of your life hasn't even begun! The point I want to make is no matter how young or old you think or know you are (just between you and me, age means absolutely nothing), you are never too young or old to be what you desire to be. And more to the point, to make changes in your body and life to make it everything it can be. Never, ever let the lies and myths that most people accept about age, and what you're supposed to do and not do, keep you from the living the life of your passions, hopes, desires and dreams.

THIS WEEK'S EXERCISE TIP

One exercise that you did in school and that the military still does today is push-ups. Depending on how you do them, push-ups will work the arms, chest and shoulders. And lucky for you, there are easy and difficult ways to it. First the easy way: Kneel down. While keeping your knees on the floor, let your upper torso come forward and spread your hands out to about shoulder-width. Push your body up until your arms are locked out. Lower your body and repeat. The next more difficult way is by keeping your legs locked out and upper and lower body in a straight line by keeping the knees off the floor and only your feet and hands touching the floor. Push your body up until your arms are locked out. Lower your body and repeat. The third and toughest way to do them is by elevating your legs higher than your head. The higher the legs, the more difficult it will be. Try using different hand

218

positions (e.g., wide, close or more forward or backward). Like many, you'll find push-ups to be an exercise you'll never outgrow.

THIS WEEK'S NUTRITION TIP

Next time you decide to splurge on a dessert and see that blueberry pie, go for it. Not only does it taste great, but it also has lots of those good things for the body called antioxidants that help the brain and body coordination. And regarding the ala mode? Okay, go ahead and have that one scoop—you deserve it.

37

The Little Things I Did This Week
To Help Me Reach My Goal and
Change My Body and Life

For Nutrition: _____

_____

_____

_____

_____

_____

_____

_____

For Exercise: _____

_____

_____

_____

_____

_____

_____

_____

The Little Things I Did This Week To Help Me Reach My Goal and Change My Body and Life

37

For Thinking Differently: _____

_____

_____

_____

_____

_____

_____

To Help Inspire Myself: _____

_____

_____

_____

_____

_____

_____

_____

37

The Little Things I Did This Week To Help Me Reach My Goal and Change My Body and Life

The Changes I Can See: _____

_____

_____

_____

_____

_____

_____

_____

The Changes I Can Feel: _____

_____

_____

_____

_____

_____

_____

_____

38
WEEK

Quote of the Week

If you deliberately plan to be less than you are capable of being, then I warn you, that you will be unhappy for the rest of your life. You will be evading your own capacities and possibilities.

—Dr. Abraham Maslow

THIS WEEK'S MENTAL TIP

Have you ever given anything less than your best effort? (C'mon, we all have.) How did it make you feel? Did it feel like you cheated yourself? When we know we are capable of giving more or being better at what we can do, then anything less than our personal best somehow sticks in our minds as less-than-happily memorable. Yet there's a fine line you would be wise to walk between doing too much and not doing enough. Take exercise, for example. You can do too much and over-train, or you can do too little and under-train; both will hold you back. The secret, if there is one, is to know what your body needs and then do it with your best efforts at that moment on that day. The reward is not only an effort well done but the powerful positive emotions that will give you the confidence to want to give your best in other areas of your life.

THIS WEEK'S EXERCISE TIP

We all have to go grocery shopping, right? Hey, who doesn't enjoy eating? Ah, but what if you could make a little mini-workout out of grocery shopping all at the same time? No problem. Whether you're buying a tub of laundry detergent, a gallon of milk or anything else that has a bit of weight to it, go ahead and pick it up and hold it longer than you normally would. Not only that, but do something like an exercise when you're holding it, like lifting it a few times up and down and out to your sides to work those shoulders. Or, flex those arms as you curl whatever you're holding up and down. Perhaps as you hold it, you quickly bend up and down a few times to work those thighs. The trick is to become more active by doing little bits of exercise here and there in the course of a day, while doing the things you'd normally do anyway.

THIS WEEK'S NUTRITION TIP

I've got a fruit for you that will keep your body healthy and... ahem... shall we say "regular" each day. It's prunes, and this little fruit is jammin' with all those great antioxidants a body needs. Try the regular and dried varieties.

38

The Little Things I Did This Week To Help Me Reach My Goal and Change My Body and Life

For Nutrition: _____

_____

_____

_____

_____

_____

_____

_____

_____

For Exercise: _____

_____

_____

_____

_____

_____

_____

_____

_____

The Little Things I Did This Week
To Help Me Reach My Goal and
Change My Body and Life

38

For Thinking Differently: _____

_____

_____

_____

_____

_____

_____

_____

_____

To Help Inspire Myself: _____

_____

_____

_____

_____

_____

_____

_____

_____

38

The Little Things I Did This Week
To Help Me Reach My Goal and
Change My Body and Life

The Changes I Can See:

_____

_____

_____

_____

_____

_____

_____

_____

The Changes I Can Feel:

_____

_____

_____

_____

_____

_____

_____

_____

39

WEEK

Quote of the Week

Know the three big lies: What I don't have is better than what I've got. More is always better. I'll be happy when I finally get what I want.

—Anonymous

THIS WEEK'S MENTAL TIP

The three big translations for this week's quote:

1. The grass is rarely greener on the other side.

2. The more things you have, the more they will own you and your life.

3. You'll be happy when you give up the need to be happy.

THIS WEEK'S EXERCISE TIP

If you take a shower each day, then it's time we put a little zest in your body—and I'm not talking soap. Think of it: doing a neat little workout to get that lower back and those abs in better shape, all while enjoying a nice, warm shower to relax and soothe the rest of your body. It's the best of both worlds, I tell you! We'll start with lower back. Simply turn away from the showerhead and put a slight bend to the knees (the legs don't need to be completely locked out) and bend over with your upper body and let your fingers touch the tub underneath you. Bring the upper body up until it's straight up and own and do it again and again until you've done it 15-20 times. To work the abs, turn around and face the showerhead. Keep your body erect with feet standing firmly. Raise your arms and hold them close to your body and in front of you. Now start twisting from side to side and do this for 1-2 minutes without stopping. Start off slowly and you'll find you'll be able to increase your range of motion and your side-to-side speed in no time.

THIS WEEK'S NUTRITION TIP

Be careful of the vitamin robbers. While scientists and research tell us that drinking (wine in particular) in moderation has beneficial health effects, alcohol can also rob the body of B vitamins, so go easy. And I needn't have to mention this, but if you're still smoking (right now is the best time to stop) or if you're exposed to secondhand smoke at home, at work or in restaurants, then you might want to increase your vitamin C intake. Research suggests that just one cigarette destroys about 25 mg of vitamin C, which would be the amount in about half a medium size orange.

39

The Little Things I Did This Week
To Help Me Reach My Goal and
Change My Body and Life

For Nutrition: _____

_____

_____

_____

_____

_____

_____

_____

_____

For Exercise: _____

_____

_____

_____

_____

_____

_____

_____

_____

The Little Things I Did This Week
To Help Me Reach My Goal and
Change My Body and Life

39

For Thinking Differently:

_____

_____

_____

_____

_____

_____

_____

_____

To Help Inspire Myself:

_____

_____

_____

_____

_____

_____

_____

_____

_____

39

The Little Things I Did This Week To Help Me Reach My Goal and Change My Body and Life

The Changes I Can See: _____

_____

_____

_____

_____

_____

_____

_____

The Changes I Can Feel: _____

_____

_____

_____

_____

_____

_____

_____

40
WEEK

Quote of the Week

You were born an original. Don't die a copy.

—Anonymous

THIS WEEK'S MENTAL TIP

Stop for a moment and be thankful for just one thing: being who and what you are right now. I couldn't care less about the terrific person you're *going* to be once you do this or achieve that. It doesn't matter to me what you look like, how young or old or how wise or unwise you think you are. All that matters is who you are, right now: the person who is reading this. Your life and appearance can change quickly and easily, so that's no big deal. Who I'm admiring and whom I want you to admire, perhaps for the first time in a long time, as you look into your mirror before you go to bed tonight, is the one-of-a-kind original masterpiece that's you. Who you are, who you will become and your life are your gifts. How you use them, for the short time you have on this earth, is your gift to yourself and to others. Never sacrifice your gift for anything or anyone.

THIS WEEK'S EXERCISE TIP

We talked about shower exercises last week, and now it's time for a bath. These two bathtub exercises will work the abs and stretch out that stiff lower back after a hard day's work. First the abs. Lie down in the tub like you normally would, but bend the knees and bring them back towards your waist as you bring up the legs and feet. The feet can even touch the wall or tub wall in front of you, if you'd like some support. This is almost the same position you'd be in if you were doing a crunch (similar to a sit-up). Now bring the upper torso up and forward towards the knees and hold it there for 1-2 seconds and then bring it back down and repeat. Do this for 12-25 times. When finished, keep those legs up where they are; and this time, with both hands, grab your knees or ankles, and pull them back towards your upper body. Feel it stretch your lower back. Bring the legs back far enough until you can feel a nice stretch in that lower back area, and hold it in that position for 4–6 seconds; then release. (Remember, we want no pain, just a stretch that feels, oh, so good to that lower back.) Do it three more times just like that.

THIS WEEK'S NUTRITION TIP

People spend billions of dollars each year on skin products, but so many of them are getting it wrong. Instead of spending all that money and time taking care of the outside, they'd be surprised how much money they'd save if they took care of the inside first. And when it comes to your skin, that means eating a healthy, balanced diet of fresh and nutritious foods and drinking lots of water to hydrate those cells. It also means getting enough vitamin A to keep skin smooth, getting enough vitamin B to keep skin looking young and firm and enough vitamin C to keep it pliable, elastic and resistant to infection.

40

The Little Things I Did This Week To Help Me Reach My Goal and Change My Body and Life

For Nutrition: _____

_____

_____

_____

_____

_____

_____

_____

_____

For Exercise: _____

_____

_____

_____

_____

_____

_____

_____

_____

The Little Things I Did This Week
To Help Me Reach My Goal and
Change My Body and Life

40

For Thinking Differently: _____

_____

_____

_____

_____

_____

_____

_____

To Help Inspire Myself: _____

_____

_____

_____

_____

_____

_____

_____

40

The Little Things I Did This Week
To Help Me Reach My Goal and
Change My Body and Life

The Changes I Can See:

_____

_____

_____

_____

_____

_____

_____

The Changes I Can Feel:

_____

_____

_____

_____

_____

_____

_____

41
WEEK

Quote of the Week

There are two things to aim at in life: first, to get what you want; and, after that, to enjoy it. Only the wisest of mankind achieve the second.

—Logan Pearsall Smith

THIS WEEK'S MENTAL TIP

Here's what I want you to do at the end of this week and every week you read this book. Take five minutes to recall the little things you did during that week to build a new body and new you. If you did that one extra rep on a tough exercise, give yourself a pat on the back. If you ate only two scoops of ice cream instead of the usual three, then smile. If you parked farther away from the mall, school or work, just so you could walk for a bit more exercise, then let yourself feel good for a job well done. You see, all those little things are the very things that will make a big difference. By themselves, they may not seem like much, but when you multiply them together, along with all the other little things you did that week, then very quickly and with very little effort, you set in motion powerful forces that change bodies and lives in big ways. Each and every week, take a few minutes to enjoy where you are and how far you've come, and to get excited about next week and all the great things that will happen in your life.

THIS WEEK'S EXERCISE TIP

One of the toughest things you'll have to do is pull yourself back from working out, especially when you're making such great progress, but it's essential that you do. Many people keep exercising, day in and day out, year after year, with too little to show for their efforts except perhaps, a body that looks the same, is fast approaching burnout (especially if they've done lots of high-intensity training) and is in a rut. Far too many people find out when it is too late that if they had treated their bodies better and given themselves the rest the needed, they could have avoided being injured and maintained their motivation. These mandatory rest breaks will help you stay injury-free and avoid the pitfalls and frustration of burnout and little or no progress. Keep your body refreshed and renewed, and you will be ready, willing and able for your next workout schedule. When should you take some time off? I recommend *taking at least one full week off from training every 4-6 weeks*. That means, every month and a half, you're going to rest and do nothing but give your body a rest. Go on "workout vacation"; relax, do nothing but enjoy yourself. You're going to find that by taking a full week off every 4-6 weeks, your body will be in a state of progressive results. That is, week after week, your body will be improving during that 4-6 week cycle of training. Taking a week off, while your body is still in that progressive-results cycle, will put you in control; you will be the one who has allowed it to stop at that higher level, and it will be from there that you will resume when you begin your next 4-6 week cycle of training. Think of it as if your body is on a continuous uphill road: Each one-week period you take off allows your body to pause at a rest stop along the way; and when you return after that week off to train again, your body gets back on the road uphill to the next rest stop.

THIS WEEK'S NUTRITION TIP

I've found a delicious and nonfat ice cream treat you can quickly make yourself. Take a sliver of your favorite nonfat frozen yogurt or ice cream. Spread it on two of your favorite flavored rice cakes (such as blueberry or chocolate or any other flavor) and make a sandwich. Place it in the freezer for at least 30 minutes and eat. Yum... great taste and no fat!

41

The Little Things I Did This Week To Help Me Reach My Goal and Change My Body and Life

For Nutrition: _____

_____

_____

_____

_____

_____

_____

_____

_____

For Exercise: _____

_____

_____

_____

_____

_____

_____

_____

_____

**The Little Things I Did This Week
To Help Me Reach My Goal and
Change My Body and Life**

41

For Thinking Differently: _____

_____

_____

_____

_____

_____

_____

_____

To Help Inspire Myself: _____

_____

_____

_____

_____

_____

_____

_____

_____

41

The Little Things I Did This Week To Help Me Reach My Goal and Change My Body and Life

The Changes I Can See: _____

_____

_____

_____

_____

_____

_____

_____

The Changes I Can Feel: _____

_____

_____

_____

_____

_____

_____

_____

42
WEEK

Quote of the Week

We do not stop playing because we grow old; we grow old because we stop playing.

—Anonymous

THIS WEEK'S MENTAL TIP

I want you to quit working out... if... it ever becomes unenjoyable. Listen. Exercising should be fun and enjoyable if you expect to make it a part of your life; and if it hasn't been fun and enjoyable in the past, it's time we change that right now. The first thing to know that will make you happier is the fact you actually need very little time to exercise to get really good results. Only a few minutes in some cases, so throw away the belief that you must do lengthy workouts or lots of sets and exercises—you simply don't need them. Just that right there should take some of the guilt and pressure off you and make things more fun. Next, it's no big deal if you miss a workout here and there, or if your diet goes to heck in a hand basket. Just start back where you left off, and you'll be fine. Now are you starting to smile? Good! You see, working out and all the other things in your life are much more meaningful when they're fun. When you can look forward to doing them, you begin to be excited like a kid, all over again. That's when your life gets back to making you happy. As they say, life is much too important to be taken seriously. Make each day your day to laugh, play and enjoy.

THIS WEEK'S EXERCISE TIP

One of the best exercises I've found for the legs is one you can do at home, and all you need is your body and a wall. They're called *Wall Deep Knee Bends,* and they work great. Think of doing these just like doing a squat, only with no weight. In essence, all you're really doing is keeping your upper body erect and bending at the knees and squatting up and down. Where you place your feet will affect, to some degree, where you feel the exercise. Legs close and feet pointed straight ahead and you'll most likely feel it in the overall quad (the front of the legs above the knees), and this should help give your legs the appearance of a nice outer sweep. Feet turned out and away from the body will tend to place the emphasis on the inner thighs. Legs and feet turned further out and away from the body—like a ballet-type stance—shift more work on the inner and upper/inner thigh. Regardless of the position of your legs and feet, always make sure your knees travel in a straight line over your toes. To really make the quads burn, try doing these deep knee bends with your back against a wall. This will add resistance to the exercise and help you maintain strict form and will definitely make the legs work harder. Try to go down to the parallel position and do non-stop, non-lockout (where the legs are bent and not 90° straight up and down) reps for even better results.

THIS WEEK'S NUTRITION TIP

Let me give you a little tip to remember that has worked well for lots of people: Too many carbs will make you drowsy, and too much protein will keep you awake. Now use that tip if you're planning for a big meeting and you need to be mentally sharp by eating some extra protein like low-fat/nonfat yogurt, cottage cheese, skim milk or half a sandwich of turkey breast or chicken on whole wheat. Likewise, if you've had a million things on your mind and you're pretty amped up and want to power down, try eating some extra carbs, like a small plate of pasta and a scoop or two of low-fat/nonfat frozen yogurt/ice cream.

42

The Little Things I Did This Week To Help Me Reach My Goal and Change My Body and Life

For Nutrition: _____

_____

_____

_____

_____

_____

_____

_____

For Exercise: _____

_____

_____

_____

_____

_____

_____

_____

The Little Things I Did This Week To Help Me Reach My Goal and Change My Body and Life

42

For Thinking Differently: _____

_____

_____

_____

_____

_____

_____

_____

To Help Inspire Myself: _____

_____

_____

_____

_____

_____

_____

_____

42

The Little Things I Did This Week
To Help Me Reach My Goal and
Change My Body and Life

The Changes I Can See: _____

_____

_____

_____

_____

_____

_____

_____

The Changes I Can Feel: _____

_____

_____

_____

_____

_____

_____

_____

43

WEEK

Quote of the Week

Never build a case against yourself.

—Robert Rowbottom

THIS WEEK'S MENTAL TIP

One question and you've got to give a quick answer: Whenever you think about trying something new, is it easier for you to give more reasons why you *can* do it or why you *can't*? How did you answer? If you hesitated and wanted to say you could think of more reasons why you could do it, but knew it wasn't true, then welcome to a big fan club. Forget having enemies, people simply don't need them when they've got the toughest foe they'll ever face staring back at them in the mirror. Next time you're out in public, listen to what people say to each other. You'll be amazed to hear just how negative, self-defeating and deflating the things are that people tell each other and themselves about themselves. Truly, if you say over and over again what your limitations are, how quickly they become true. Tell yourself the good stuff instead!

THIS WEEK'S EXERCISE TIP

I know you probably wouldn't think so, but simply by moving the elbows up or down, or into the body or away, can affect how an exercise feels. Let's take the dumbbell kickback for the triceps. Most people will do this exercise with their working upper arm either close to their body or hanging down below their body. Wrong. The trick is to keep the upper arm close to the body but make it come up *above* the upper body. Try this and you'll see. Do a dumbbell triceps kickback, and the higher you raise the working elbow and dumbbell above your body, the tougher this exercise will get.

THIS WEEK'S NUTRITION TIP

Time to get rid of that nasty LDL (low-density lipoprotein) cholesterol with some great foods that you probably have in the pantry or refrigerator but may not have known about. Here are two easy ones: oat bran and oatmeal. Other good ones are beans, barley, grapefruit, skim milk, garlic, onions, eggplant, olive oil, apples, oranges, carrots and yogurt.

43

The Little Things I Did This Week
To Help Me Reach My Goal and
Change My Body and Life

For Nutrition: _____

_____

_____

_____

_____

_____

_____

_____

_____

For Exercise: _____

_____

_____

_____

_____

_____

_____

_____

_____

_____

The Little Things I Did This Week
To Help Me Reach My Goal and
Change My Body and Life

43

For Thinking Differently:

_____

_____

_____

_____

_____

_____

_____

_____

To Help Inspire Myself:

_____

_____

_____

_____

_____

_____

_____

_____

43

The Little Things I Did This Week To Help Me Reach My Goal and Change My Body and Life

The Changes I Can See: _____

_____

_____

_____

_____

_____

_____

_____

_____

The Changes I Can Feel: _____

_____

_____

_____

_____

_____

_____

_____

_____

44
WEEK

Quote of the Week

When you get into a tight place and everything goes against you, till it seems as though you could not hold on a minute longer, never give up then, for that is just the place and time that the tide will turn.

—Harriet Beecher Stowe

THIS WEEK'S MENTAL TIP

Something I've found to be a source of inspiration is how much things and people's lives can change in 24 hours. One day, it could be the last straw in a series of events we thought we could no longer take; and then the next day, the good news comes in and changes everything in a flash. The hardships are gone and the good times have arrived. The same is true of exercise and diet. It may seem like weeks will go by and you will have put all that time and work into doing all the right things; and yet little, if any, progress comes your way. Then a few days later, your eyes open to the new changes you now begin to see taking shape in your body. Those few extra pounds that just wouldn't come off now seem to have finally disappeared. And it's all because you hung in there when you felt like giving up. Yes, when you've reached the end of your rope and don't want to go on any longer, that's the point when the good stuff is going to happen for you. It's amazing the difference just another day or two makes.

THIS WEEK'S EXERCISE TIP

Some weeks back, I talked to you about push-ups and what a terrific exercise it is. Well, here's another way to do them—that will work chest and triceps—and it's standing up facing a wall. Keeping your body erect, stand about 12-24 inches away from a wall. Place your hands on the wall—hands spaced wide hits more chest, and hands closer works more triceps—and let your body come forward toward the wall and then push it back out to the starting position and repeat. Don't allow your body to bend as it comes forward; keep it straight. Go for 6-12 reps or until you feel a burning sensation in the muscles.

THIS WEEK'S NUTRITION TIP

Now lets' raise that good HDL (high-density lipoprotein) cholesterol with such things as raw onions, olive oil and wine (go for the red variety); and, of course, keeping your diet low fat will really help.

44

The Little Things I Did This Week
To Help Me Reach My Goal and
Change My Body and Life

For Nutrition: _____

_____

_____

_____

_____

_____

_____

_____

_____

For Exercise: _____

_____

_____

_____

_____

_____

_____

_____

_____

The Little Things I Did This Week To Help Me Reach My Goal and Change My Body and Life

44

For Thinking Differently: _____

_____

_____

_____

_____

_____

_____

_____

_____

To Help Inspire Myself: _____

_____

_____

_____

_____

_____

_____

_____

_____

44

The Little Things I Did This Week To Help Me Reach My Goal and Change My Body and Life

The Changes I Can See:

_____

_____

_____

_____

_____

_____

_____

_____

_____

The Changes I Can Feel:

_____

_____

_____

_____

_____

_____

_____

_____

_____

45
WEEK

Quote of the Week

Sometimes it is more important to discover what one cannot do than what one can do. So much restlessness is due to the fact that a man does not know what he wants, or he wants too many things, or perhaps he wants to be somebody else, to be anybody except himself.

–Lin Yutang

THIS WEEK'S MENTAL TIP

I've heard it said that in our lives, we can have anything; it's just we can't have everything. There's a big difference. We simply aren't given enough years to have everything there is to have. But, for the things we deeply desire, we can most definitely have them if we'll do what's required to make them our own. Make no mistake, we each have talents and abilities that allow us to do things easier than others, just as others have their talents and abilities that allow them to do other things easier than we can. Each person has different talents and callings in life, and the wisest of us are the ones who listen to that calling and follow it. The problem, it seems, comes when we don't know what we want or we think we'll have forever to do whatever it is we finally decide to do, whatever it may be. The truth is, we don't have unlimited time to use our unlimited desires. You, I and everyone else are given the same 1,440 minutes each day, and we each have only a certain number of years to make the most of each of those days. Each day you choose not to follow your dream is one less day you'll have for enjoying it. Follow the voice of your calling and begin it today.

THIS WEEK'S EXERCISE TIP

An old proverb says, "The person who does not find time for exercise will have to find time for illness." This speaks volumes about how important exercise is to your life. From the age of the Greeks to Thomas Jefferson's time, it was believed that a simple walk (one that doesn't fatigue you) was the best single exercise anyone could do. Even today, few would argue. The Greeks also believed that life was movement; and that the more movement they did, the more the life force would course through their bodies and the better they would feel and the longer they would live. So, don't sweat it if you have no time for a gym, no time for a proper workout with machines, weights and the like. Simply do more walking. Walk anywhere and everywhere you can; and along with that, make your body move more. When doing your daily tasks, move those arms and legs more than you normally would, and do it often.

THIS WEEK'S NUTRITION TIP

We all like junk food every now and then. What works great for a lot of people is to eat a good diet for six days and on the seventh day relax and have those junk foods they've been craving And to really give your body the disease-fighting and life-sustaining nutrients it needs (the phytochemicals), try eating more foods that have been shown to help the body prevent disease, such as peppers, red beets, citrus fruit, onions, garlic, bok choy, Brussels sprouts, grapes, broccoli, cabbage, mustard greens, cauliflower, leeks, carrots, apples, rutabaga, chives, collards, turnip greens, kale, kohlrabi and tomatoes.

45

The Little Things I Did This Week To Help Me Reach My Goal and Change My Body and Life

For Nutrition: _____

_____

_____

_____

_____

_____

_____

_____

For Exercise: _____

_____

_____

_____

_____

_____

_____

_____

The Little Things I Did This Week To Help Me Reach My Goal and Change My Body and Life

45

For Thinking Differently: _____

_____

_____

_____

_____

_____

_____

_____

To Help Inspire Myself: _____

_____

_____

_____

_____

_____

_____

_____

42

The Little Things I Did This Week
To Help Me Reach My Goal and
Change My Body and Life

The Changes I Can See: _____

_____

_____

_____

_____

_____

_____

_____

The Changes I Can Feel: _____

_____

_____

_____

_____

_____

_____

_____

46

WEEK

Quote of the Week

All through history we find convincing proof that mental powers increase with age, that artistic and intellectual powers are often intensified in later years. Michelangelo was still producing masterpieces at eighty-nine. Goethe completed the second part of Faust when he was eighty-two. Wagner finished Parsifal at sixty-nine, and Voltaire wrote Candide at sixty-five. Handel was still composing beautiful music, Longfellow was still writing immortal poetry, after seventy.

—Lillian Eichler Watson

THIS WEEK'S MENTAL TIP

"The older you get, the wiser you become" is a maxim that's just as true today as it was hundreds of years ago. And with that wisdom comes the realization that when one decides to become masterful at anything in life, age doesn't matter. The point is to decide to be great at something, be it raising a family or creating a work of art. Each is equally valuable and needed. Many times we think it advantageous that others started their quest to greatness at such an early age, only later to find out that those we admired are miserable because they give up some many precious years of their youth in order to become so great. And, for many of them, if they had it to do all over again, they would've waited and experienced more of life and living and allowed their genius to unfold and develop without such all-or-nothing drive and determination to be first, and while still being young. Whatever your age and whatever your experience, right now is the best time to begin your quest to greatness, be it a refreshed body, heart and soul or new direction in your life.

THIS WEEK'S EXERCISE TIP

Let's face it: In the course of an average day, especially at school or at the office, you might not have time to do the exercises you'd like to, out of apprehension of what others might say if they saw you. Oh, but here's a stealthy little exercise that works your abs that no one will know you are doing. Stand or sit. With your upper body erect, using your normal breathing rhythm, breathe out, then take a deep breath in—as big a breath in as possible—and hold it for 1-2 seconds. Blow that big (not bad) breath out and do it again. Do this up to 10 times, two or three times a day, for a cool little stomach toner.

THIS WEEK'S NUTRITION TIP

One of the cheapest, easiest and tastiest ways to help keep your body feeling good is by eating wheat bran each day. And all you need is just one cup of your favorite wheat bran cereal to do it.

46

The Little Things I Did This Week To Help Me Reach My Goal and Change My Body and Life

For Nutrition: _____

_____

_____

_____

_____

_____

_____

_____

_____

For Exercise: _____

_____

_____

_____

_____

_____

_____

_____

_____

_____

The Little Things I Did This Week
To Help Me Reach My Goal and
Change My Body and Life

46

For Thinking Differently: _____

_____

_____

_____

_____

_____

_____

_____

_____

To Help Inspire Myself: _____

_____

_____

_____

_____

_____

_____

_____

_____

46

The Little Things I Did This Week To Help Me Reach My Goal and Change My Body and Life

The Changes I Can See: _____

_____

_____

_____

_____

_____

_____

_____

_____

The Changes I Can Feel: _____

_____

_____

_____

_____

_____

_____

_____

_____

47

WEEK

Quote of the Week

A man may have a home, possessions, a charming family, and yet find all these things ashy to his taste because he has been outstripped in the marathon race by some other runners to the golden tape line. It is not that he does not possess enough for his wants but that others possess more. It is the more that haunts him, makes him deprecate himself, and minimizes his real achievements... The time has come when a man must say to himself: "I am no longer going to be interested in how much power or wealth another man possesses so long as I can attain enough for the dignity and security of my family and myself.

I am going to break through this vicious circle which always asks the question of life in a comparative degree: 'Who is bigger?' 'Who is richer?' 'Who has more?' I am going to set my goals for myself rather than borrow them from others. I will strive to achieve a mature attitude toward success which is ambition for growth and accomplishment, real accomplishment rather than spurious, decorative, and vanity-filled acquisition. I refuse any longer to destroy my peace of mind by striving after wind, and I will judge myself in the scale of goodness and culture as well as in the balance of silver and gold." Such a man is on the road to avoiding the neurotic materialism of our age. He is like the poet who does not tear himself to pieces because his sonnet is not equal to that of Shakespeare. He is like the musician who does not always despise his little fugue because it lacks the magic of Bach. He is like the poet or musician who learns to accept himself and be happy with his own growth from year to year rather than paralyze his gifted pen or his talented ear by contrast with the giants and the immortals... only when we harness our own creative energies to goals which are of our own adult choice, not imposed upon us by the compulsions of unresolved childhood competition, can we call ourselves mature and happy.

—Joshua Loth Liebman

277

THIS WEEK'S MENTAL TIP

The body and life you've been given is not an eternal challenge to be forever unhappy and always wanting to change. You can have no desire to change how you look and feel and be as happy as those who do. It's all about what you desire to make different in your life and why. Have you allowed yourself to be sucked into the competitive vibe and allowed that to be your guide to what you should do next? Or have you instead unlocked those chains and decided to live your life and look and feel the way you do because that's exactly what you want, without a care as to what others think? If you're the latter, then congratulations, for you are on the road to living happy, living well. We don't need to prove anything to anyone but ourselves. With or without change, with or without success, you are just as awesome—and you don't need anyone to tell you otherwise.

THIS WEEK'S EXERCISE TIP

Here's a wonderful series of quick and easy exercises you can do anywhere or anytime you want, that will help keep you flexible, increase range of motion and are terrific de-stressors. The first is for the wrists. Hold the right wrist with the left hand and freely move the right hand in a big circle from left to right, right to left. Repeat for the other hand. Now do the same kind of movement for the ankles. You can either sit down and hold the one ankle with the other hand and do it or while standing, lift the leg off the ground and move the foot in a circle from right to left and left to right. And now for a great de-stressor for the head and neck: Slowly begin turning your head from left to right. Do this for 8-10 times. Next, allow the head to relax and let it hang down as you turn it slowly and gently from side to side. Finally, while being relaxed, begin slowly turning your head in a relaxing circle and do this for six times to right, then six times to the left. Relax and feel the stress and tension evaporate from your body each time your head moves.

THIS WEEK'S NUTRITION TIP

Things are going to get a little fishy here. Time for some fish tips. Number one: Try having fish 1-3 times a week. Number two: Go for the smaller or younger fish since they have fewer years and chances of being exposed to chemicals and pollutants than bigger or older fish . Number three: Freshwater salmon or trout is good, but you might want to lean more on saltwater fish than other freshwater fish (Many believe that bigger bodies of water reduce the potential ill effects of pollution and absorption by fish). Number four: try cooking fish—either on the grill or in the oven—by placing it in aluminum foil, basted with a light coating of extra virgin olive oil and sprinkled with basil or rosemary leaves over it, plus a good squeeze of lemon juice. Cover it completely and cook at 300-350° for 20 minutes. Unwrap, serve, and simply throw away the wrapper. No mess or smell, and almost effortless.

47

The Little Things I Did This Week To Help Me Reach My Goal and Change My Body and Life

For Nutrition: _____

_____

_____

_____

_____

_____

_____

_____

For Exercise: _____

_____

_____

_____

_____

_____

_____

_____

_____

The Little Things I Did This Week To Help Me Reach My Goal and Change My Body and Life

47

For Thinking Differently:

_____

_____

_____

_____

_____

_____

_____

_____

To Help Inspire Myself:

_____

_____

_____

_____

_____

_____

_____

_____

47

The Little Things I Did This Week To Help Me Reach My Goal and Change My Body and Life

The Changes I Can See: _____

_____

_____

_____

_____

_____

_____

_____

The Changes I Can Feel: _____

_____

_____

_____

_____

_____

_____

48
WEEK

Quote of the Week

*If a man does not keep pace with his companions,
perhaps it is because he hears a different drummer.
Let him step to the music which he hears,
however measured or far away.*

—Henry David Thoreau

THIS WEEK'S MENTAL TIP

You might begin an exercise program or different diet and it could be the one that's the latest buzz or the bestseller everyone is following, and yet it doesn't do anything for you. Not following it any longer is the very best thing you could do. So many people out there are like sheep that need a shepherd to guide them to the next pasture, but you are not like them. Regardless of your experience, inside you is an unfailing inner knowing that knows what works and what doesn't in your life. Follow it wherever it leads you and do whatever you are led to do, to have the body and life you know can be yours. You're much smarter and wiser than you may think.

THIS WEEK'S EXERCISE TIP

You've been doing great all these weeks, trying lots of the different exercises and tips I've been giving you, so it's time for a sleep tip. After all, sleep is at least as important to the body as exercise. This one's easy: Get rid of the alarm clock. That's right, take it out of your bedroom and watch how much better you'll sleep at night. Oh sure, at first you may be a bit hesitant, since you may have come to depend on it each day to wake you in time. However, if you'll trust your own body clock to awaken you, you won't be disappointed. Try either covering up the clock or unplugging it on the weekends and allow your body to awaken naturally. Notice how it makes you feel. After a few weekends of getting used to no clock, try doing without it on one day during the week, perhaps a day you normally go in later. Before you know it, you'll be waking within minutes before the time you set on the alarm. Trust your instincts and allow your mind and body to guide you. You're about to be amazed at how much more restfully you'll sleep and how much better you'll feel when you awaken.

THIS WEEK'S NUTRITION TIP

If you want your body to be a lean machine, here's some good advice to follow: As the day gets later, reduce the amount of carbohydrates while keeping the protein intake consistent. Many believe the body's insulin is more active earlier in the day than in the evening. And if the body's ability to use and move insulin is lower at night, it suggests a greater likelihood that those great-tasting, late-night carbohydrate snacks could be more easily stored as fat.

48

The Little Things I Did This Week To Help Me Reach My Goal and Change My Body and Life

For Nutrition: _____

_____

_____

_____

_____

_____

_____

_____

For Exercise: _____

_____

_____

_____

_____

_____

_____

_____

The Little Things I Did This Week
To Help Me Reach My Goal and
Change My Body and Life

48

For Thinking Differently: _____

_____

_____

_____

_____

_____

_____

_____

To Help Inspire Myself: _____

_____

_____

_____

_____

_____

_____

_____

48

The Little Things I Did This Week To Help Me Reach My Goal and Change My Body and Life

The Changes I Can See: _____

_____

_____

_____

_____

_____

_____

_____

The Changes I Can Feel: _____

_____

_____

_____

_____

_____

_____

_____

49
WEEK

Quote of the Week

Before we set our hearts too much upon anything, let us examine how happy they are who already possess it.

—Francois de La Rochefoucauld

THIS WEEK'S MENTAL TIP

My goodness, how we think we'd be so much happier if we only could have more time, money, success or anything else we don't already have in our lives. We look at envy with the woman who's thin and shapely or the guy who has model looks and a body to match. But little do we realize or understand the whole picture. Speaking from experience, I can tell you that I've known many women and men who *had all the beauty you could ask for, but had all the problems you'd never want.* While much of their lives were focused on the physical, far less of it was devoted to the mental and spiritual; and once you got beyond the outer shell, you could immediately sense the void on the inside. Sure, you'd like to change a few things in your life, try something new or get rid of things that aren't working any longer, and I know you'll do it. But on the way to doing those things, let yourself be happy for who you are right now. Perhaps your life isn't so bad after all.

THIS WEEK'S EXERCISE TIP

So, how do you know when you're making progress? The first way is to ask yourself, "How do I feel?" If you're feeling better about yourself and your body, then you're doing something right and making progress. The next step would be to accurately assess how you look. And don't use the scale to do it. If you put too much emphasis on achieving a certain number—as in losing or gaining weight (remember the majority of scales tell you how much weight and not *fat* that you've lost)—then much of how you feel about yourself and your progress will be tied into what the scale tells you. The scale can be a real liar at times, since it doesn't tell you the changing composition of your body, but only a number of how much it weighs. As you know, muscle weighs more than fat, so if your body is changing and losing the fat and adding a bit of lean, healthy muscle tissue, you can actually be looking and feeling better and weighing more. But, if you are just paying attention to how much you weigh, then the added weight might really bum you out and steal your motivation, and you will lose your inspiration to keep working out. To get a good indication of how your body is changing (and it will change, believe me), then use a mirror. The mirror doesn't care how much you weigh. It simply reflects back to you, what you look like at that given moment of the day. And your body can change greatly from hour to hour and day to day, due to hormones, sleep, food and fluid intake, water retention, etc. So if you must look in the mirror, then try doing it at different times on different days to see how your body changes. The other feedback method—and one I prefer—is to use a pair of old tight fitting pants. If you're still having problems getting them on, then you've got a bit more work to do. If the pants are getting easier to slip on or getting loose, then you're on the right track. Be careful of using just any kind of pants, especially jeans that have just been washed and dried; they can shrink up and make you think you're heavier than you really are.

THIS WEEK'S NUTRITION TIP

If you occasionally have trouble falling asleep, try eating a light snack that has sugar or honey on it. Stay away from the high-fat cookies and snacks. Instead, try eating a bagel or rice cake with a nice spread of honey and see if that does the trick.

49

The Little Things I Did This Week To Help Me Reach My Goal and Change My Body and Life

For Nutrition: _____

_____

_____

_____

_____

_____

_____

_____

_____

For Exercise: _____

_____

_____

_____

_____

_____

_____

_____

_____

The Little Things I Did This Week To Help Me Reach My Goal and Change My Body and Life

49

For Thinking Differently: _____

_____

_____

_____

_____

_____

_____

_____

To Help Inspire Myself: _____

_____

_____

_____

_____

_____

_____

_____

49

The Little Things I Did This Week To Help Me Reach My Goal and Change My Body and Life

The Changes I Can See: _____

_____

_____

_____

_____

_____

_____

_____

The Changes I Can Feel: _____

_____

_____

_____

_____

_____

_____

_____

50

WEEK

Quote of the Week

All that is necessary to break the spell of inertia and frustration is this: Act as if it were impossible to fail. This is the talisman, the formula, the command of right-about-face which turns us from failure towards success.

—Dorothea Brande

THIS WEEK'S MENTAL TIP

This quote has been a source of power and inspiration so many times in my life. Think of it: Act as if it were impossible to fail! Just what would you attempt if you knew you couldn't fail? Just what kinds of changes would you make in mind, body and spirit if you knew success was guaranteed? Just what kind of business would you open if financial and emotional success was waiting for you? William James, the Harvard scholar and philosopher, paraphrased all of this beautifully when he said, "Act as if, and you will soon become." See yourself and act as if you are the greatest success and as if it is impossible for you to fail. You will soon see just how true that will be.

THIS WEEK'S EXERCISE TIP

I like this exercise for strengthening and toning the lower back because it's quick and easy and you can do it at home. Not much movement is needed from this exercise to really work, tone and strengthen your lower back. Simply lie down with your stomach touching the floor. Keep your legs and feet close together. Place your arms and hands under your upper legs, with your hands turned so that your palms are touching the floor. Slowly raise your upper body a few inches off the floor until you can feel your lower back working. Hold your body in this a-few-inches-off-the-floor position for 1-2 seconds and then slowly lower it back down and repeat. Be sure and do slow, continuous-tension reps and you won't need to do more than 5-9 per set and only 2-3 sets.

THIS WEEK'S NUTRITION TIP

Here are a few cooking and food storage tips to make your life easier:

1. Keep your cereal in the refrigerator; it'll last longer.

2. When broiling food, add ½–1 cup of water before cooking; the water keeps the smoke away and sops up the grease.

3. To keep that pot of spaghetti, rice or noodles from boiling over, add a tablespoon of cooking oil to the water.

4. To keep cheese from getting all funky and moldy, next time try storing it in a glass jar, or else wrapped in waxed paper and then optionally stored in a zip-lock bag.

50

The Little Things I Did This Week To Help Me Reach My Goal and Change My Body and Life

For Nutrition: _____

_____

_____

_____

_____

_____

_____

_____

For Exercise: _____

_____

_____

_____

_____

_____

_____

_____

_____

The Little Things I Did This Week
To Help Me Reach My Goal and
Change My Body and Life

50

For Thinking Differently: _____

_____

_____

_____

_____

_____

_____

To Help Inspire Myself: _____

_____

_____

_____

_____

_____

_____

_____

50

The Little Things I Did This Week To Help Me Reach My Goal and Change My Body and Life

The Changes I Can See: _____

_____

_____

_____

_____

_____

_____

_____

_____

The Changes I Can Feel: _____

_____

_____

_____

_____

_____

_____

_____

_____

51
WEEK

Quote of the Week

Nobody grows old merely by living a number of years. We grow old only by deserting our ideals. Years may wrinkle the skin, but to give up enthusiasm wrinkles the soul… Whether seventy or sixteen, there is in every being's heart the love of wonder, the sweet amazement at the stars and the star-like things and thoughts, the undaunted challenge of events, the unfailing child-like appetite for what next, and the joy and game of life. You are as young as your faith, as old as your doubt; as young as your self-confidence, as old as your fear; as young as your hope, as old as your despair.

—Samuel Ullman

THIS WEEK'S MENTAL TIP

To be young, you must do three things. Number one: Think young, for old thoughts make old people. Number two: Be active. Number three: Live your life and forget your age.

THIS WEEK'S EXERCISE TIP

Knowing how to exercise makes it fun. Knowing how to avoid injuries makes it something you'll enjoy doing for the rest of your life. Here are the rules to remember:

Rule No. 1: Make time to warm up before, during and after training.

Rule No. 2: Go slow and steady. Use good exercise form and be consistent.

Rule No. 3: If at any time you feel something that is painful, stop immediately and don't do that exercise. (You'll be able to differentiate between good old-fashioned making-the-muscles-work kind of discomfort, which is normal, and real pain.) Stretch some more, and then try another exercise; if the pain persists, cool down and take a break.

Rule No. 4: Allow your body to rest completely and heal that injury. Even if many days have passed and you can still feel a slight twinge or ache, continue to rest. *If you feel the pain, then do not train!*

Rule No. 5: Once you have returned to 100%, begin very slowly by moving that body part with no weights. Start with a very limited range of motion, and then slowly and gradually increase the range of motion until it is pain-free and back to 100% normal.

Rule No. 6: Once it is 100% normal and you feel no pain or discomfort, begin to add a very light set of an exercise for that body part that is easy and comfortable for you to do. Focus on doing any kind of exercise that allows for the freest range of motion and one that will allow you to find the right and best feeling exercise groove for you and your body.

Rule No. 7: Next workout, add another weight set of that exercise. Each workout, slowly add another weight exercise until you're back to the level you had before the injury. Add weight, sets, reps and exercises slowly, and stop *immediately* if you feel *any* pain.

Rule No. 8: Include a new segment to your workout that includes more emphasis on stretching, increasing range of motion and warm-ups for any sensitive body parts/areas you might have.

Rule No. 9: *Take at least one week off from training for every 4-6 weeks of training* you do. Even if you're making great progress and feeling no injuries or pain or discomfort, take the time off. Force yourself, if you have to, to take the time off. It will do amazing things for your body, attitude and results.

THIS WEEK'S NUTRITION TIP

More and more people are looking for foods that have fewer chemicals and less processing and are more organic. Besides the taste differences, you might be surprised at the nutrition benefits when comparing organic to non-organic foods. For example, one experiment caught my eye where it was reported that organically grown potatoes had at least two times the boron and selenium and over 50% more zinc than non-organic potatoes. And organically grown wheat was equally impressive: two times the calcium, four times the magnesium, five times the manganese and thirteen times the selenium, compared to the non-organic type.

51

The Little Things I Did This Week
To Help Me Reach My Goal and
Change My Body and Life

For Nutrition: _____

_____

_____

_____

_____

_____

_____

_____

For Exercise: _____

_____

_____

_____

_____

_____

_____

_____

The Little Things I Did This Week
To Help Me Reach My Goal and
Change My Body and Life

51

For Thinking Differently:

_____

_____

_____

_____

_____

_____

_____

To Help Inspire Myself:

_____

_____

_____

_____

_____

_____

_____

_____

51

The Little Things I Did This Week To Help Me Reach My Goal and Change My Body and Life

The Changes I Can See: _____

_____

_____

_____

_____

_____

_____

_____

The Changes I Can Feel: _____

_____

_____

_____

_____

_____

_____

_____

52

WEEK

(It's been one year already; congratulations!)

Quote of the Week

Doubt whom you will, but never yourself.

—Bovee

THIS WEEK'S MENTAL TIP

When you look back on what has happened in your life and the decisions you've made and the things you've gone through as a result of those decisions, you'll start realizing something surprising. Every single thing that has happened to you, either happy or painful, has made you who and what you are today. And if you go back to an event that may have happened years ago and wonder how your life would've been different if you could erase that experience, you'll see that you can't or wouldn't want to erase it because it was the next step you needed to take that led you to the next thing that happened in your life that brought you here, where you are right now. So many times, you beat yourself up for the decisions you did or did not make, only to realize that not only did you make the best decision you could've made at that time in your life, but years later you see that going through such an experience turned out to be a huge blessing and the growing experience you needed. You have never failed and you never will fail, because you will make the best decisions you can, at the right times, on that day, and at that time in your life. Yes, the uncertainties of the economy, the events of the world and the actions of other people may cause you to doubt, but never doubt yourself, for you will always make the right decisions and you always have.

THIS WEEK'S EXERCISE TIP

Here's when it's good to be in a jamb; a doorjamb, that is. If you're ever short on time but high on enthusiasm to do at least a little something for your body, try these immovable resistance exercises that will work the arms, shoulders and chest. First, stand between a doorway or in a hallway. Place both hands on either side of you and against the doorjamb or hallway walls. Begin to push against the walls; push for 3-6 seconds, then release. Do this again for two more times. You'll feel this in the arms, chest and shoulders. Next, with arms out to your sides, place the back of the hands against the door jamb or hallway walls and do the same push for 3-6 seconds like you did before. Do this for two more times. This will work the shoulders more directly. Finally, while standing in the middle of the doorway, raise both arms above your head so the hands are touching the top of the doorway. Keep your body erect and now push the arms upward as you try to straighten them as you feel it work the shoulders. And as a bonus, if the doorway or hallway is wide enough, you can place your body with your back on one side of the doorway or against one hallway wall and place one foot on the opposite side and push your leg and hold it for 3-6 seconds against the immovable object. Do it for the other leg, and you should feel like you've had a quick little workout.

THIS WEEK'S NUTRITION TIP

This is an easy one: eat more of the foods that are good for your body, but be sure to eat the foods you enjoy. Your life is not some scientific experiment that's a test for you not to enjoy it by you cutting out the things you enjoy eating simply for the sake of seeing how long you can live. Who the heck cares how many years one lives if they haven't fully enjoyed all those years? There'll be days and times when your diet will be terrible, and other times when it will be spot on. Just do the best you can, when you can,and enjoy each day and the wonderful opportunities of choosing the foods you eat; and most of all, cherish the gift of your life.

52

The Little Things I Did This Week To Help Me Reach My Goal and Change My Body and Life

For Nutrition: _____

_____

_____

_____

_____

_____

_____

_____

_____

For Exercise: _____

_____

_____

_____

_____

_____

_____

_____

_____

The Little Things I Did This Week
To Help Me Reach My Goal and
Change My Body and Life

52

For Thinking Differently:

_____

_____

_____

_____

_____

_____

_____

_____

To Help Inspire Myself:

_____

_____

_____

_____

_____

_____

_____

_____

52

The Little Things I Did This Week To Help Me Reach My Goal and Change My Body and Life

The Changes I Can See: _____

_____

_____

_____

_____

_____

_____

_____

The Changes I Can Feel: _____

_____

_____

_____

_____

_____

_____

_____

And finally...

The Strides I Made This Past Year
To Help Me Reach My Goal and
Change My Body and Life

For Nutrition: _____

_____

_____

_____

_____

_____

_____

_____

_____

For Exercise: _____

_____

_____

_____

_____

_____

_____

_____

_____

The Strides I Made This Past Year
To Help Me Reach My Goal and
Change My Body and Life

For Thinking Differently: _____

_____

_____

_____

_____

_____

_____

_____

To Help Inspire Myself: _____

_____

_____

_____

_____

_____

_____

_____

The Strides I Made This Past Year
To Help Me Reach My Goal and
Change My Body and Life

The Changes I Can See: _____

_____

_____

_____

_____

_____

_____

_____

The Changes I Can Feel: _____

_____

_____

_____

_____

_____

_____

_____

Enjoy yourself—it is later than you think.

—Dr. Frederic Loomis

SHARE YOUR SUCCESS STORY
WITH THE WORLD

We want to hear all about your success story and how **Lose the Butt, Lose the Gut and Get Out of the Rut!** helped you achieve your success. If we choose it, you and your story could be featured in our next book.

Go to www.RobertWolff.com and click on the **Tell Me Your Story** tab for all the details.

Thank You and Best Wishes!

www.ingramcontent.com/pod-product-compliance
Lightning Source LLC
LaVergne TN
LVHW011321080426
835513LV00006B/141